THIS IS A RECORD OF MY FIRST FIVE YEARS

NAME: _____

RACHAEL HALE

MY LIFE AS A BABY

A FIVE YEAR RECORD

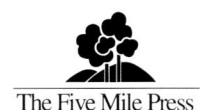

The Five Mile Press

in association with PQ Blackwell

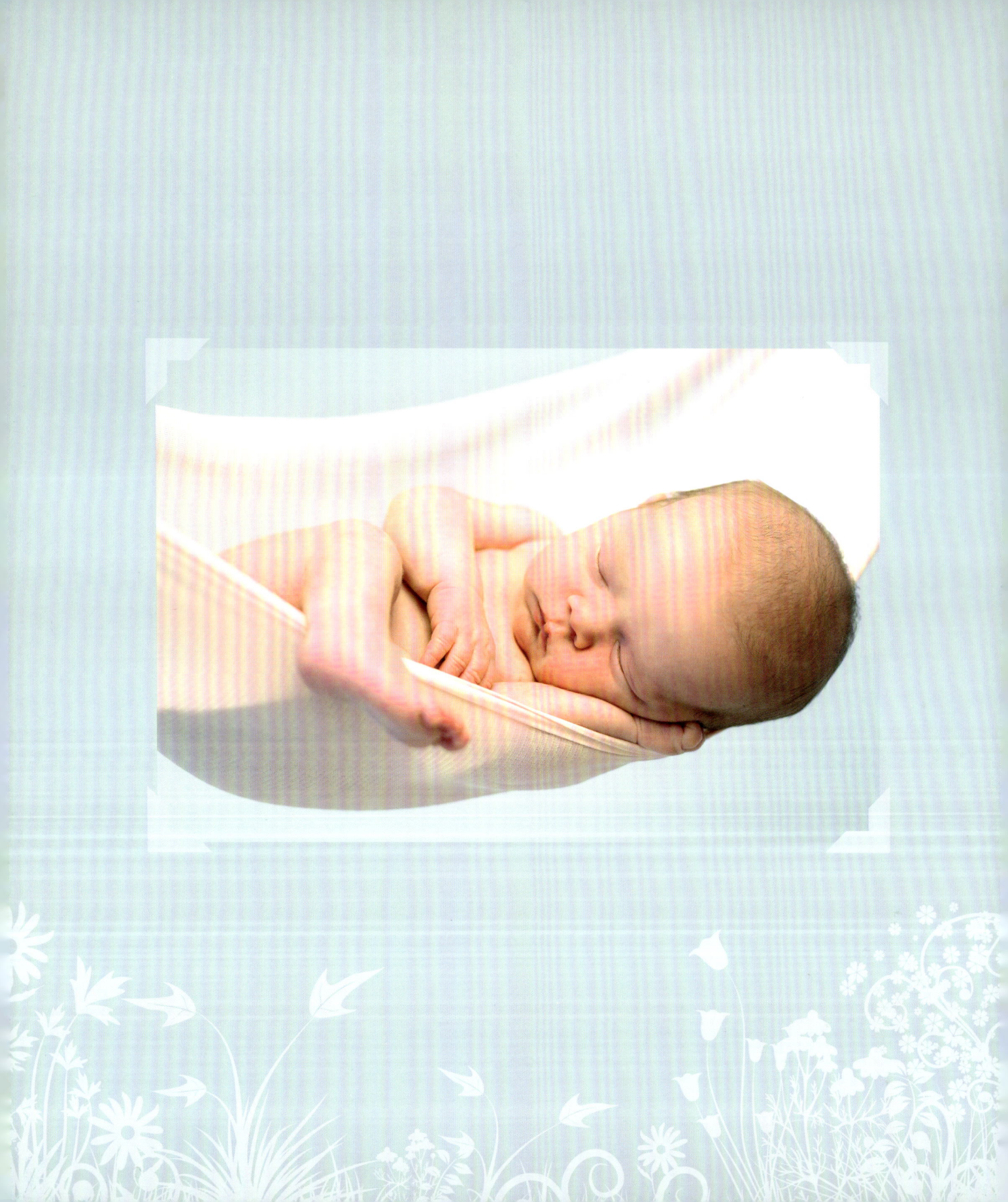

CONTENTS

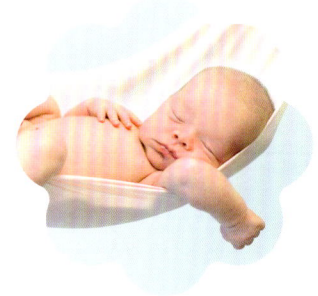

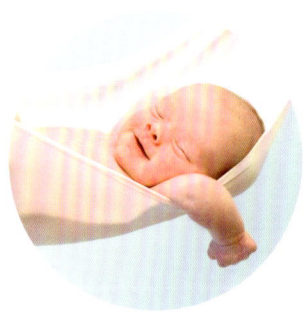

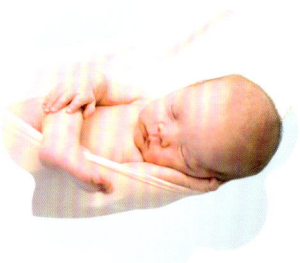

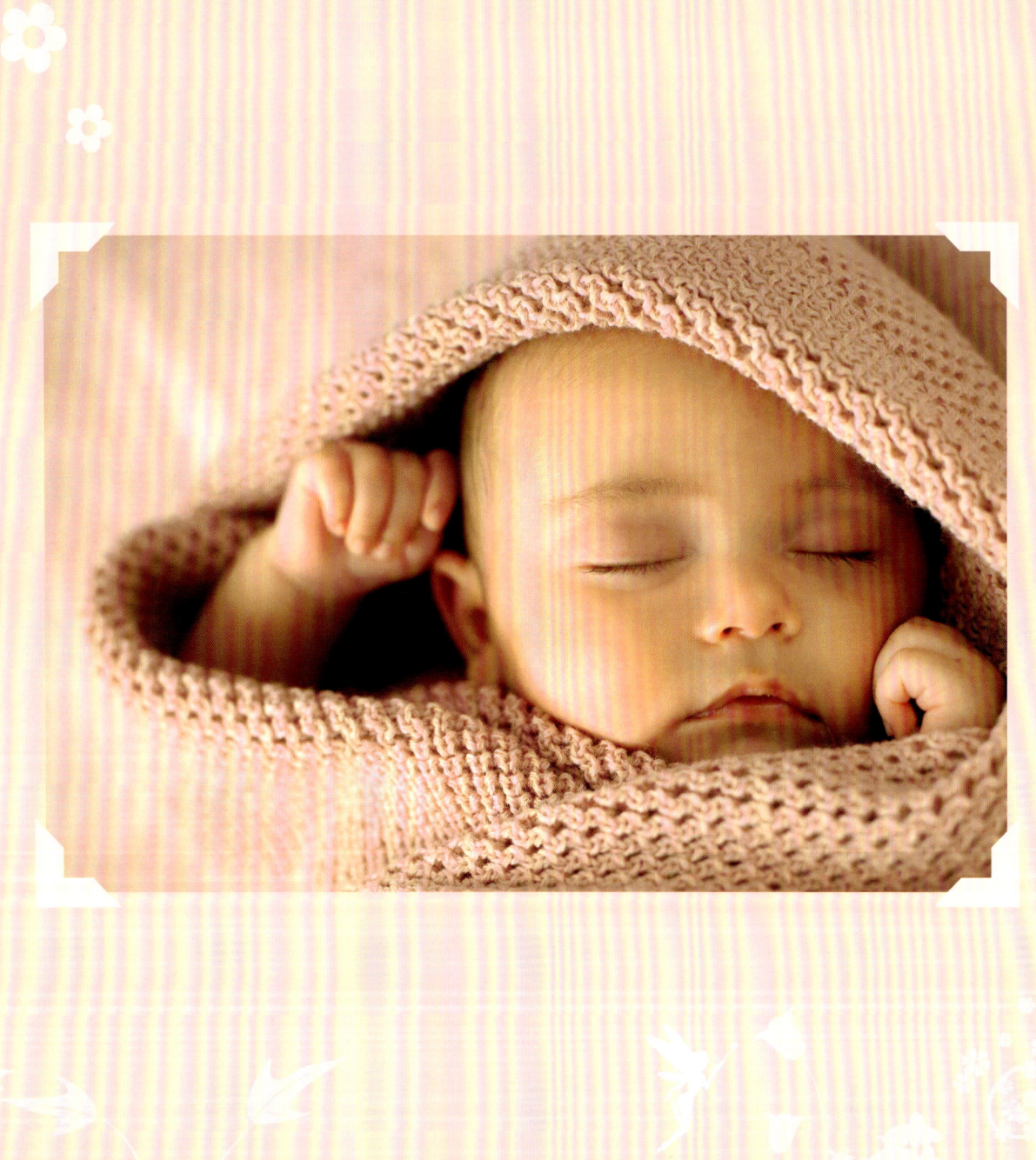

MY DUE DATE

_____

BEFORE I WAS
BORN MY PARENTS
CALLED ME

_____

_____

_____

_____

WHEN THEY WERE
EXPECTING ME MY
PARENTS FELT

_____

_____

_____

_____

_____

WHAT MY PARENTS
WERE DOING WHEN
MY MOTHER WENT
INTO LABOUR

_____

_____

_____

_____

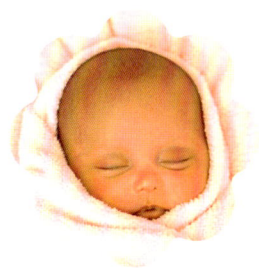

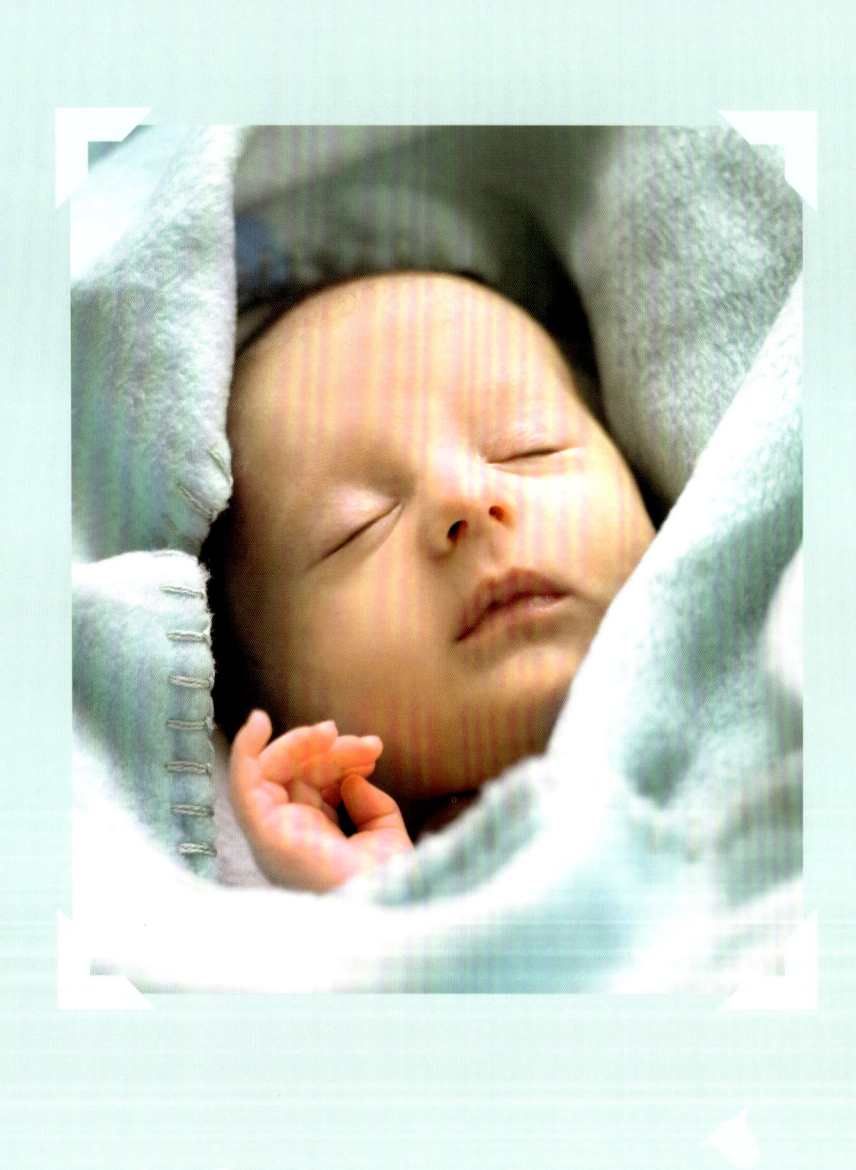

DATE

TIME

DAY OF WEEK

LENGTH OF LABOUR

LOCATION/HOSPITAL

MEDICAL TEAM

SUPPORT CREW

SPECIAL MEMORIES

YOUR PHOTO HERE

YOUR PHOTO HERE

YOUR PHOTO HERE

YOUR PHOTO HERE

PHOTOGRAPHS

YOUR PHOTO HERE

YOUR PHOTO HERE

YOUR PHOTO HERE

YOUR PHOTO HERE

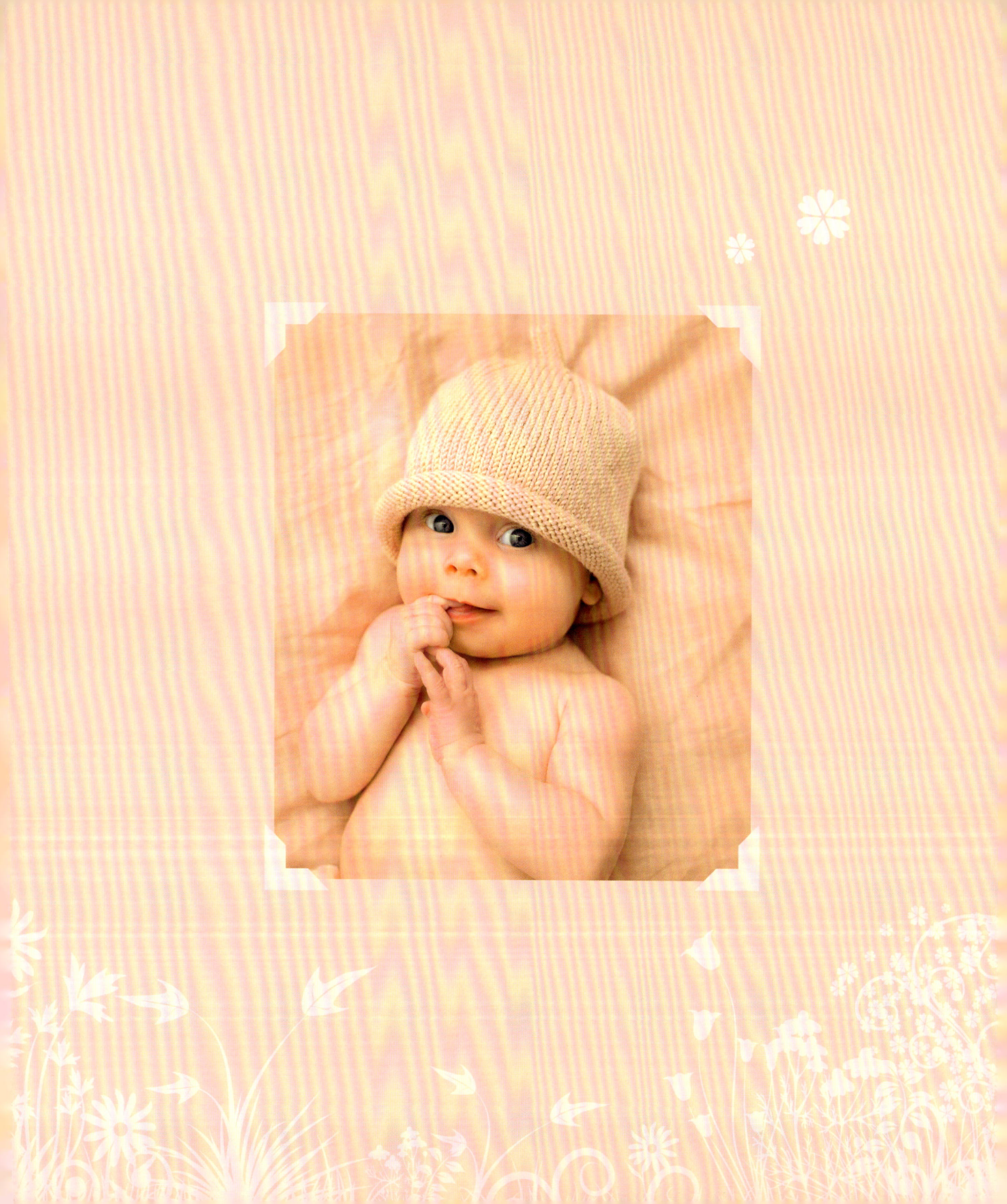

FIRST APPEARANCES

MY WEIGHT

_____

MY LENGTH

_____

MY HAIR COLOUR

_____

MY FIRST MOMENTS
WITH MY PARENTS

_____

_____

_____

_____

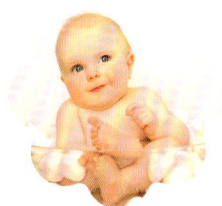

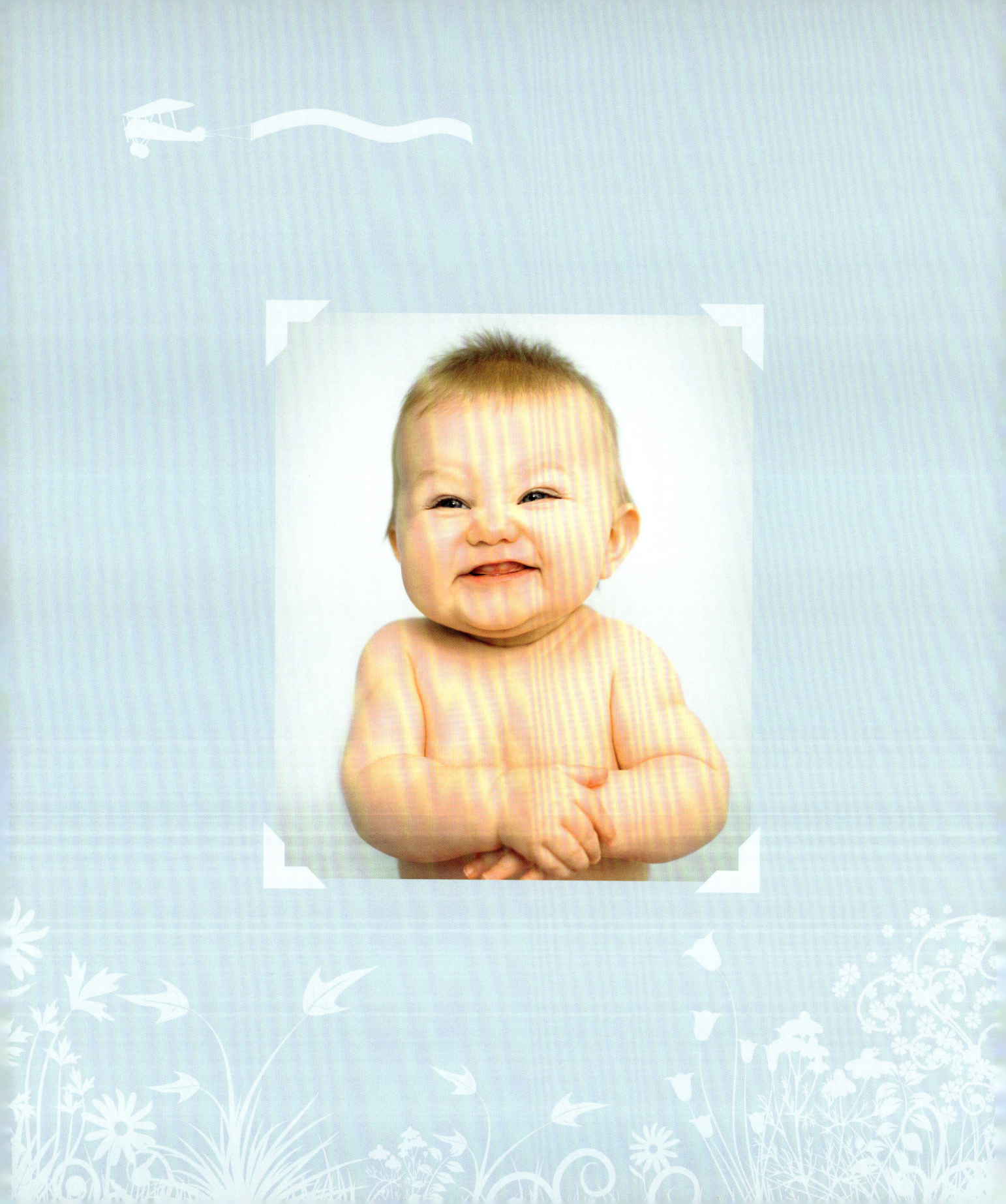

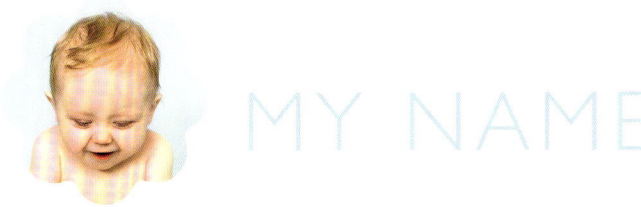

MY NAME

MY NAME IS

_____

MY PARENTS
CHOSE IT BECAUSE

_____

_____

MY NICKNAME/S ARE

_____

BECAUSE

_____

OTHER NAMES MY
PARENTS CONSIDERED
WERE

_____

_____

_____

DATE   PLACE

MY NAMING CEREMONY   _____   _____

PERFORMED BY

_____

MY CEREMONY WAS

_____

_____

MY PARENTS' FAVOURITE
MEMORY OF THE DAY

_____

_____

_____

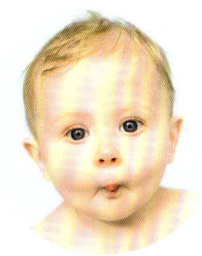

YOUR PHOTO HERE

YOUR PHOTO HERE

YOUR PHOTO HERE

YOUR PHOTO HERE

PHOTOGRAPHS

YOUR PHOTO HERE

YOUR PHOTO HERE

YOUR PHOTO HERE

YOUR PHOTO HERE

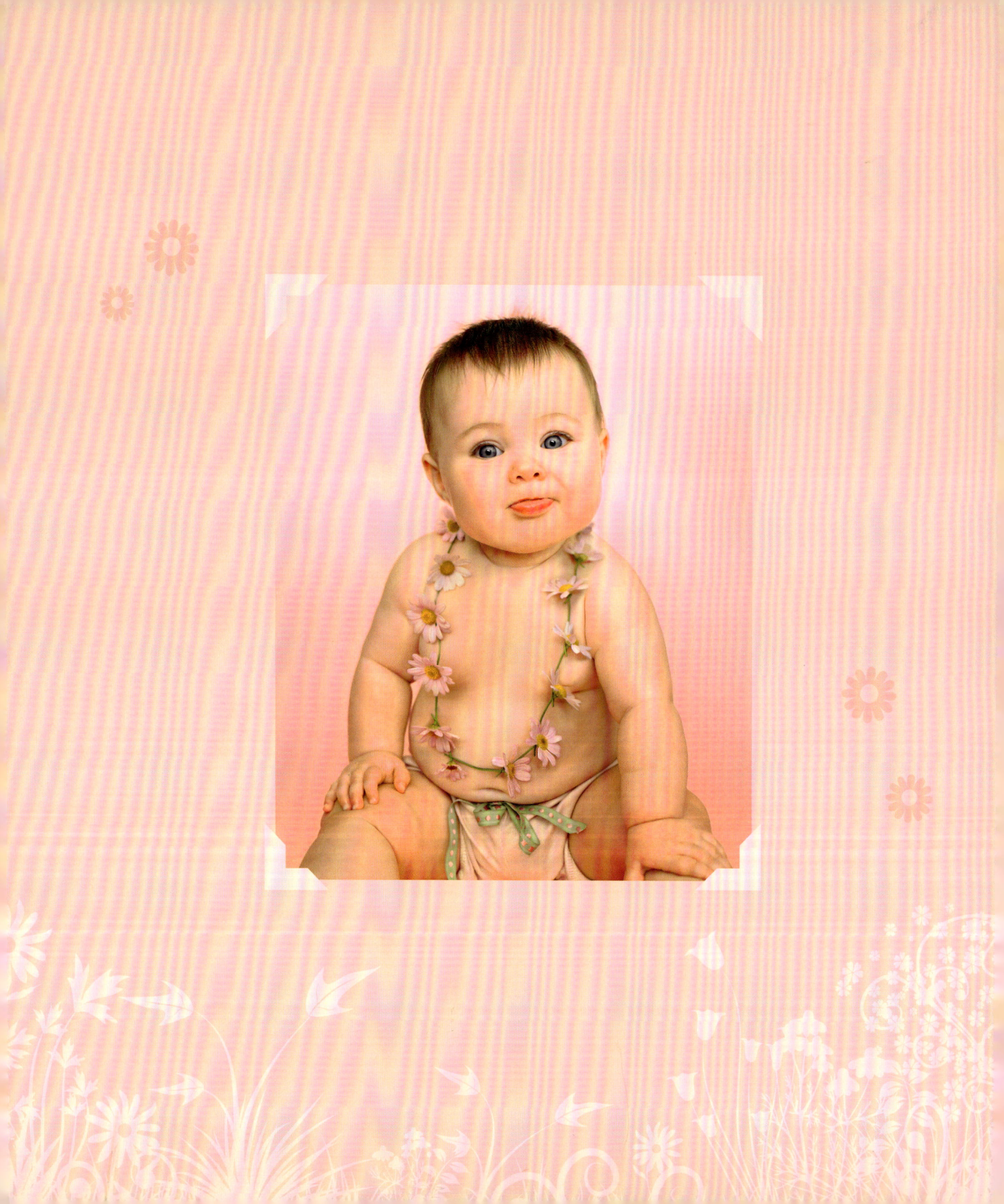

WHAT WAS HAPPENING IN THE WORLD

THE NUMBER-ONE SONG _____

THE NUMBER-ONE FILM _____

A MOVIE TICKET COST _____

ONE LITRE OF MILK COST _____

THE NEWS STORIES OF THE DAY

_____

_____

_____

_____

_____

IMPORTANT LEADERS
AROUND THE WORLD

_____

_____

_____

_____

_____

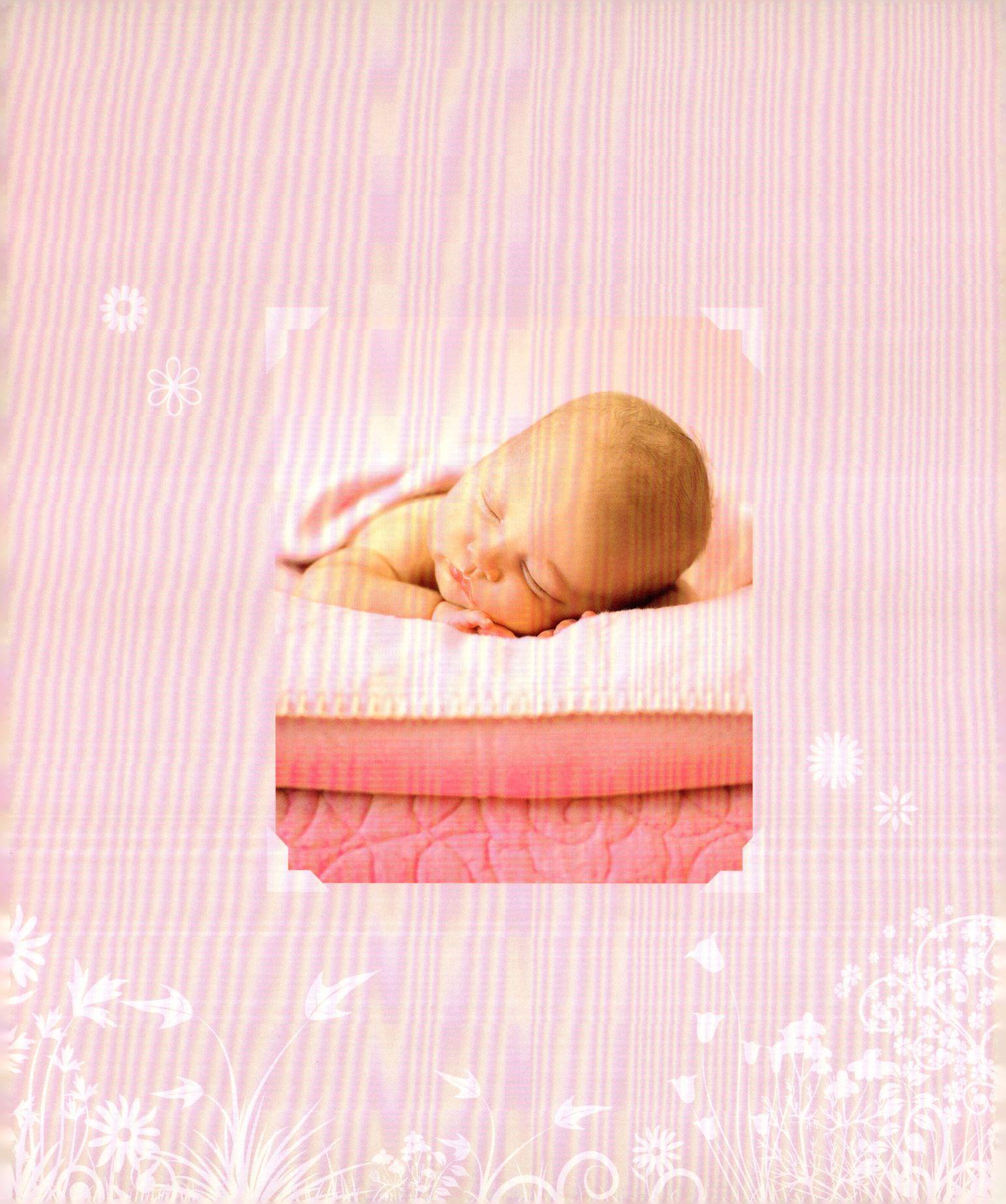

COMING HOME

MY PARENTS FELT _____

I WENT HOME ON _____

THE CAR I RODE IN WAS _____

MY FIRST HOME WAS AT _____

FAMILY AND FRIENDS
THERE TO WELCOME ME _____

_____

WHERE I FIRST SLEPT _____

I SLEPT FOR _____ HOURS

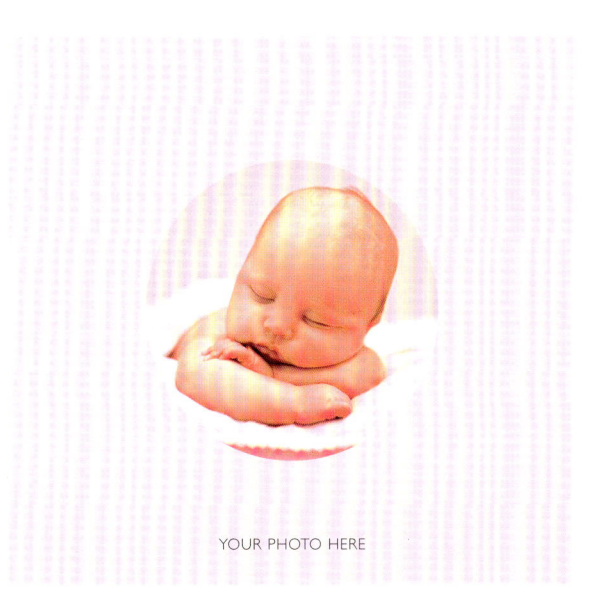

YOUR PHOTO HERE

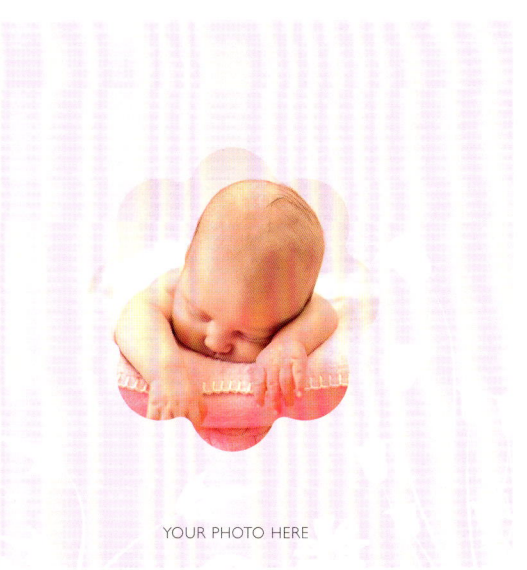

YOUR PHOTO HERE

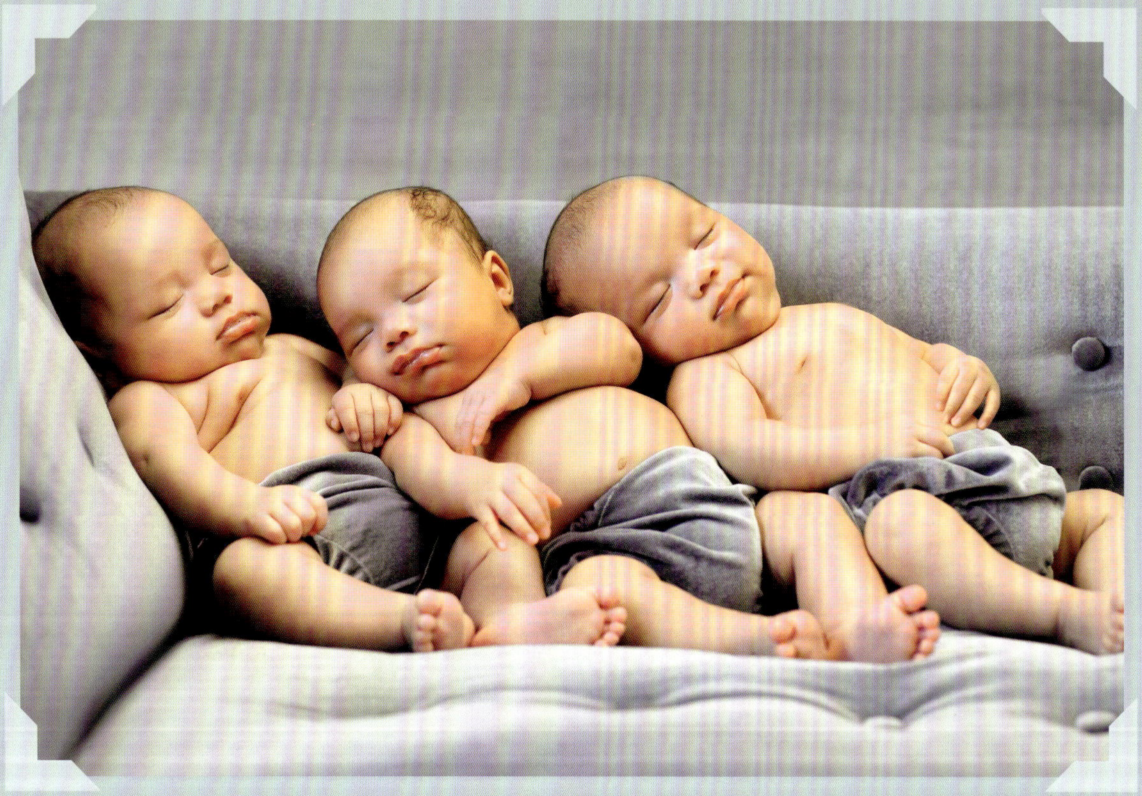

FAMILY TREE

GREAT GRANDPARENTS   GREAT GRANDPARENTS   GREAT GRANDPARENTS   GREAT GRANDPARENTS

_____   _____   _____   _____

_____   _____   _____   _____

GRANDMOTHER   GRANDFATHER   GRANDMOTHER   GRANDFATHER

_____   _____   _____   _____

AUNTS/UNCLES   MOTHER   FATHER   AUNTS/UNCLES

_____   _____

_____   _____

_____   _____

BROTHERS   ME   SISTERS

_____   _____   _____

_____   _____

_____   _____

YOUR FAMILY PHOTO HERE

YOUR FAMILY PHOTO HERE

YOUR FAMILY PHOTO HERE

YOUR FAMILY PHOTO HERE

FRIENDS & LOVED ONES

YOUR FAMILY PHOTO HERE

YOUR FAMILY PHOTO HERE

YOUR FAMILY PHOTO HERE

YOUR FAMILY PHOTO HERE

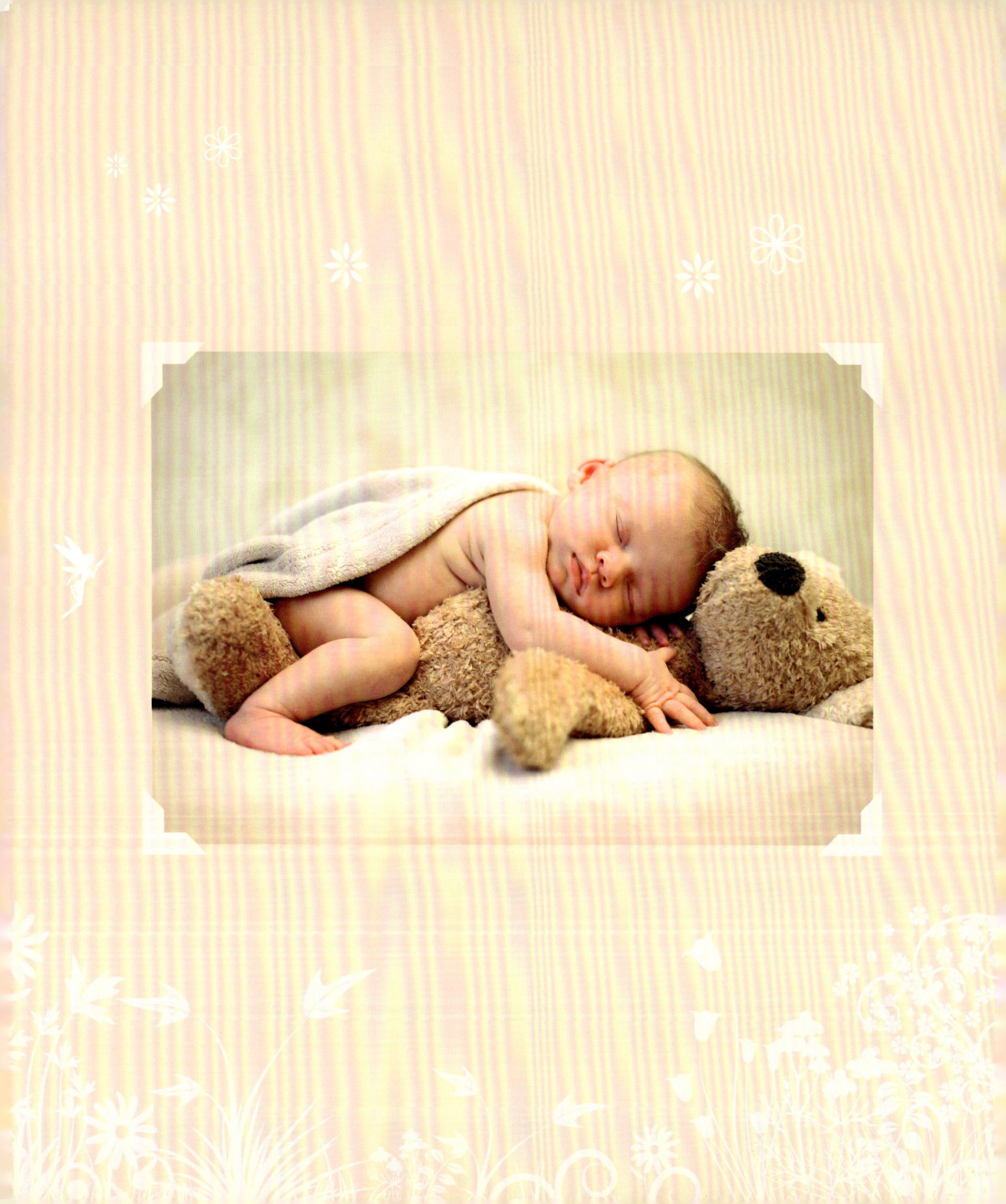

IN THE BEGINNING

_____

_____

BEDTIME RITUALS

_____

_____

_____

_____

LULLABIES I LOVE

_____

_____

_____

MY CUTEST
SLEEPING HABIT

_____

_____

_____

	AGE	DATE
IMPORTANT DATES		
SLEEPING IN A COT		
SLEEPING IN A BED		

MY FAVOURITE
BEDTIME TOY/S

_____

_____

_____

_____

PICTURE

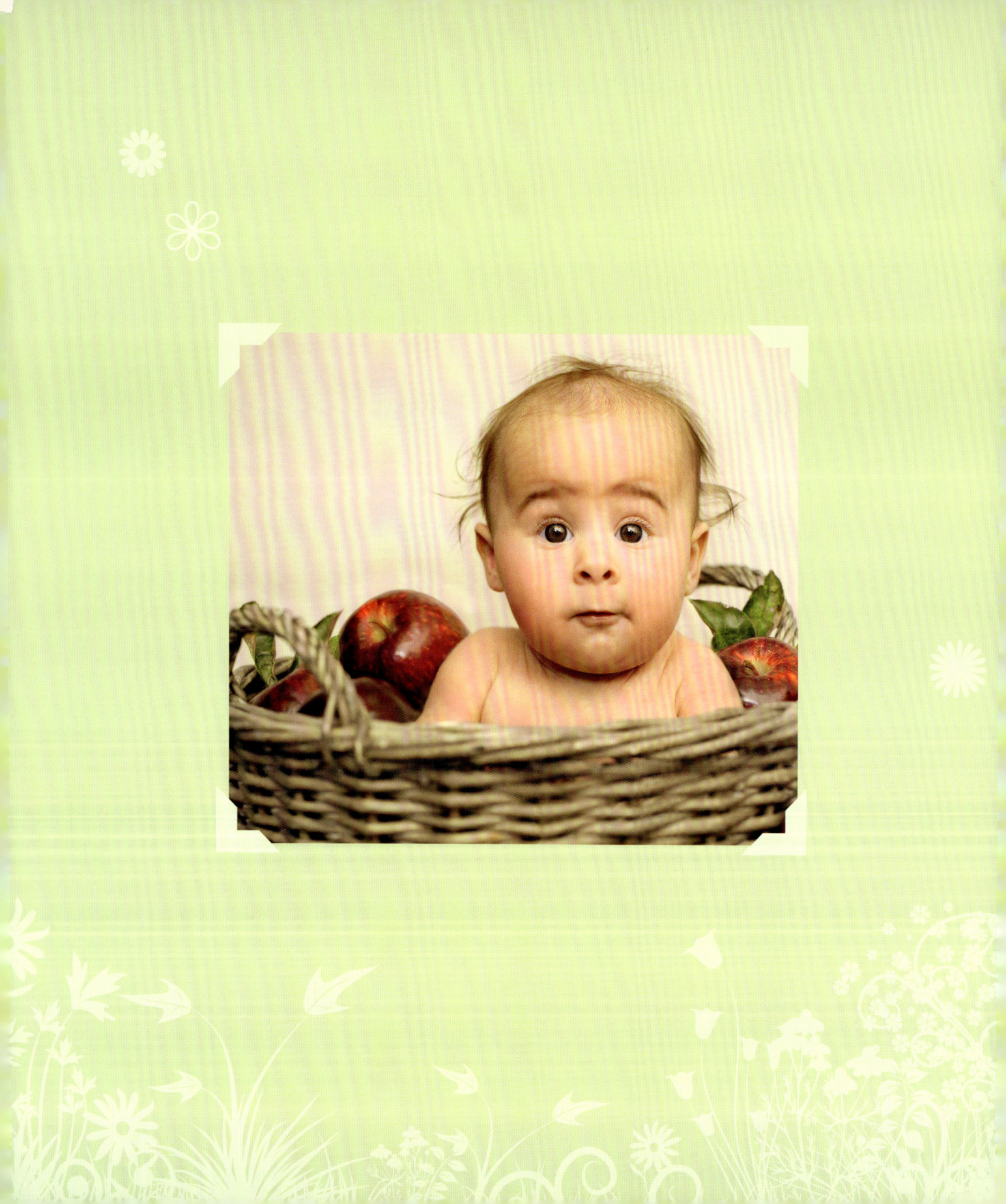

EATING

MY APPETITE

FOODS I LIKE

FOODS I DISLIKE

	AGE	DATE

WEANED FROM
BREAST/BOTTLE

MY FIRST TOOTH

EATING SOLID FOOD

SITTING IN A HIGHCHAIR

DRINKING FROM A CUP

PICTURE

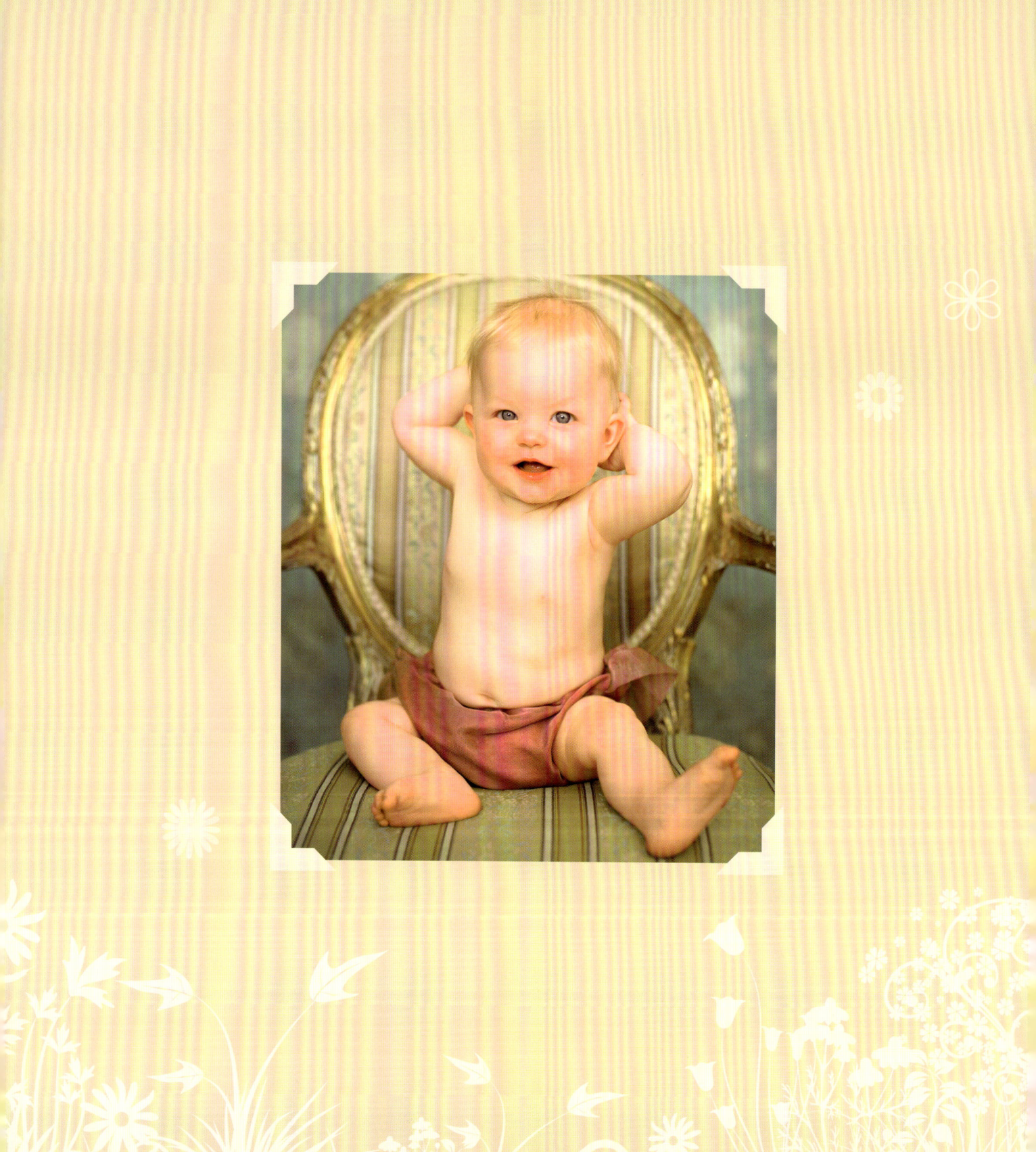

SITTING UP

AGE _____

DATE _____

CRAWLING

AGE _____

DATE _____

WAVING BYE-BYE

AGE _____

DATE _____

STANDING UP

AGE _____

DATE _____

MY FIRST STEPS

AGE _____

DATE _____

FIRST PAIR OF SHOES

AGE _____

DATE _____

SIZE _____

YOUR PHOTO HERE

YOUR PHOTO HERE

YOUR PHOTO HERE

YOUR PHOTO HERE

PHOTOGRAPHS

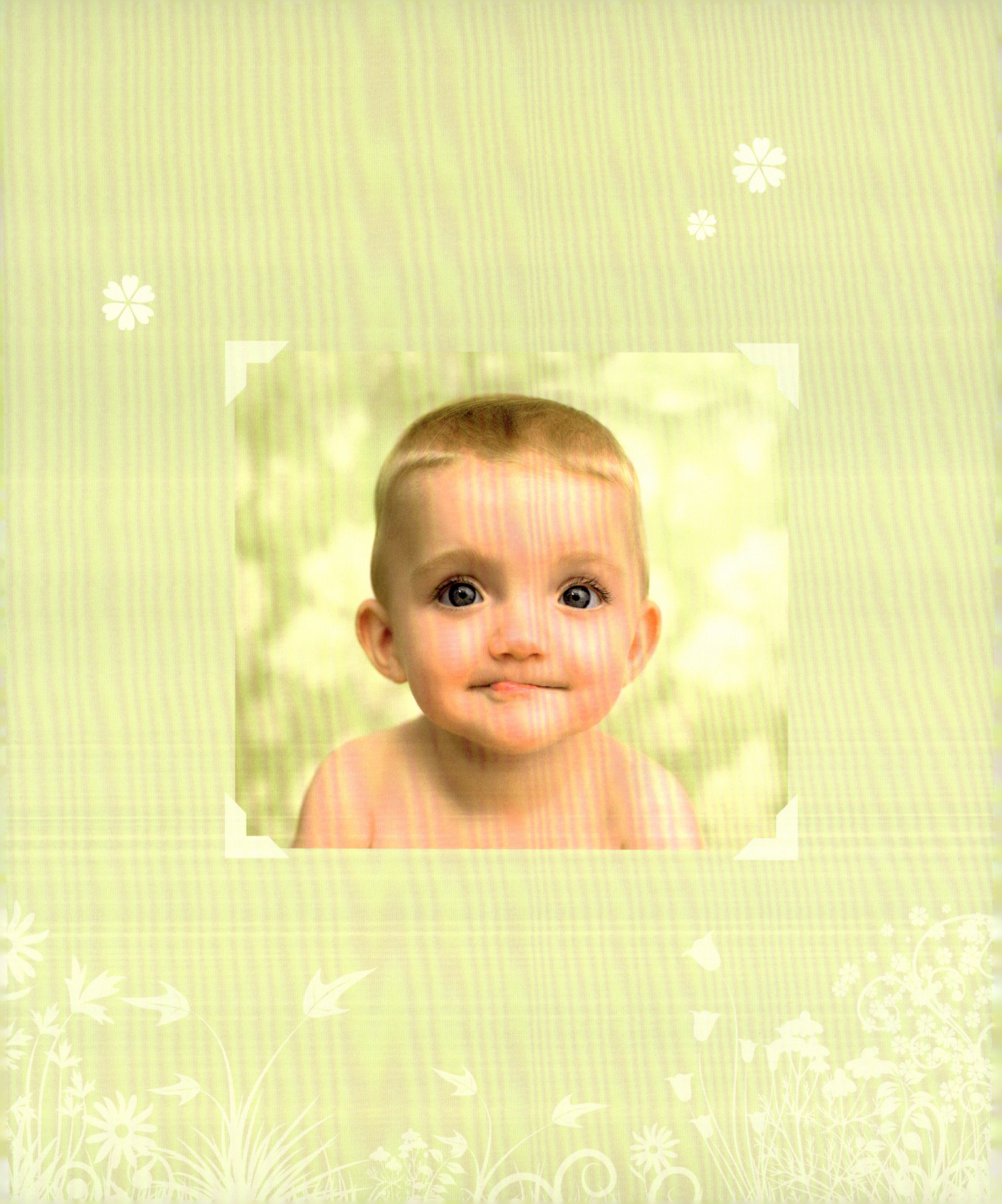

TALKING

MY FIRST WORDS

_____

_____

_____

_____

_____

MY FAVOURITE SAYING

_____

_____

_____

_____

_____

MY FAVOURITE SONG

_____

_____

_____

_____

_____

		AGE	DATE
IMPORTANT DATES	COUNTING TO TEN		
	SINGING THE ALPHABET		

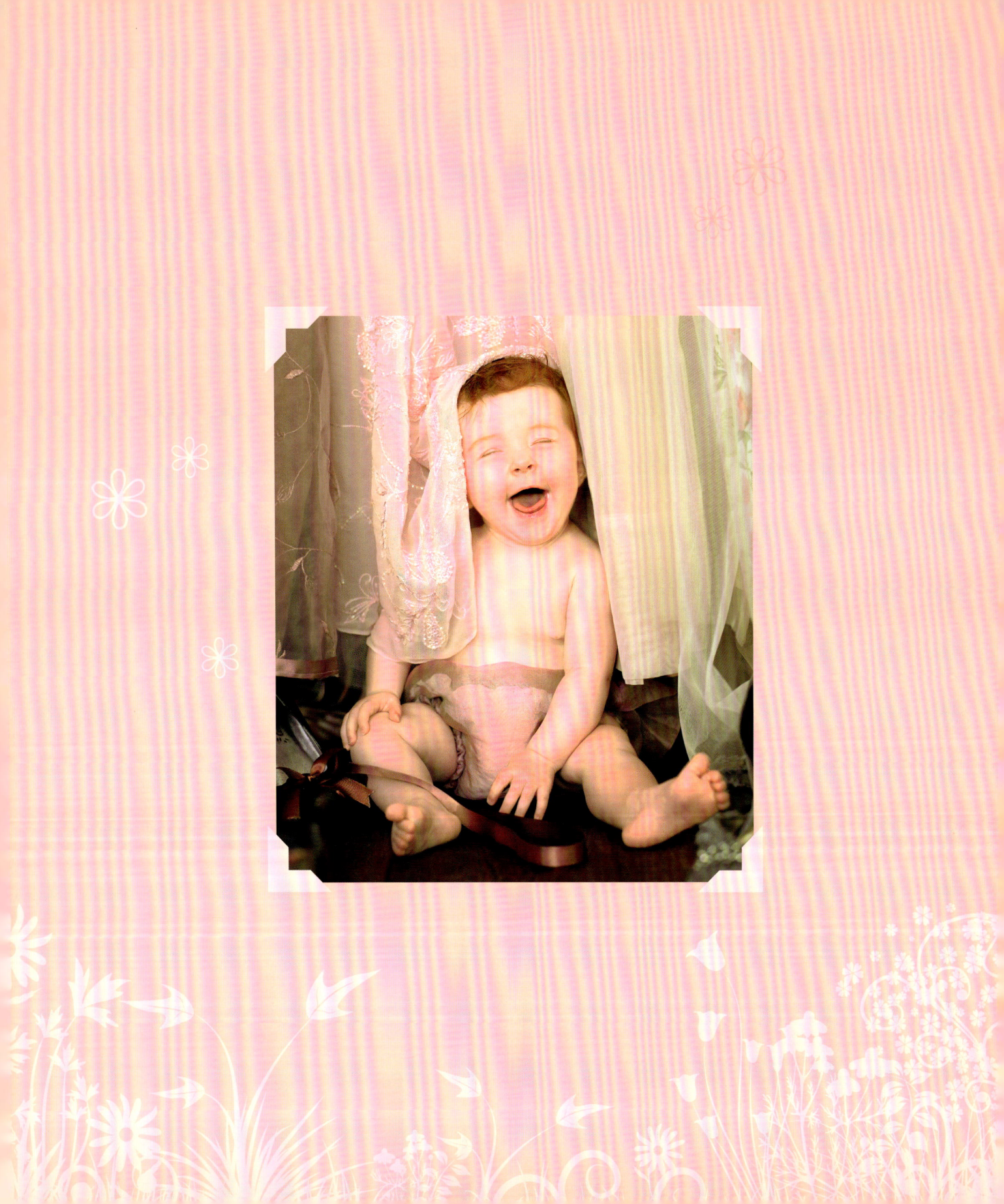

THINGS THAT MAKE ME HAPPY

_____
_____
_____
_____
_____
_____

THINGS THAT MAKE ME SAD

_____
_____
_____
_____

HOW MY PARENTS COMFORT ME

_____
_____
_____
_____
_____
_____

WHEN I WAS HAPPY

YOUR PHOTO HERE

WHEN I WAS SAD

YOUR PHOTO HERE

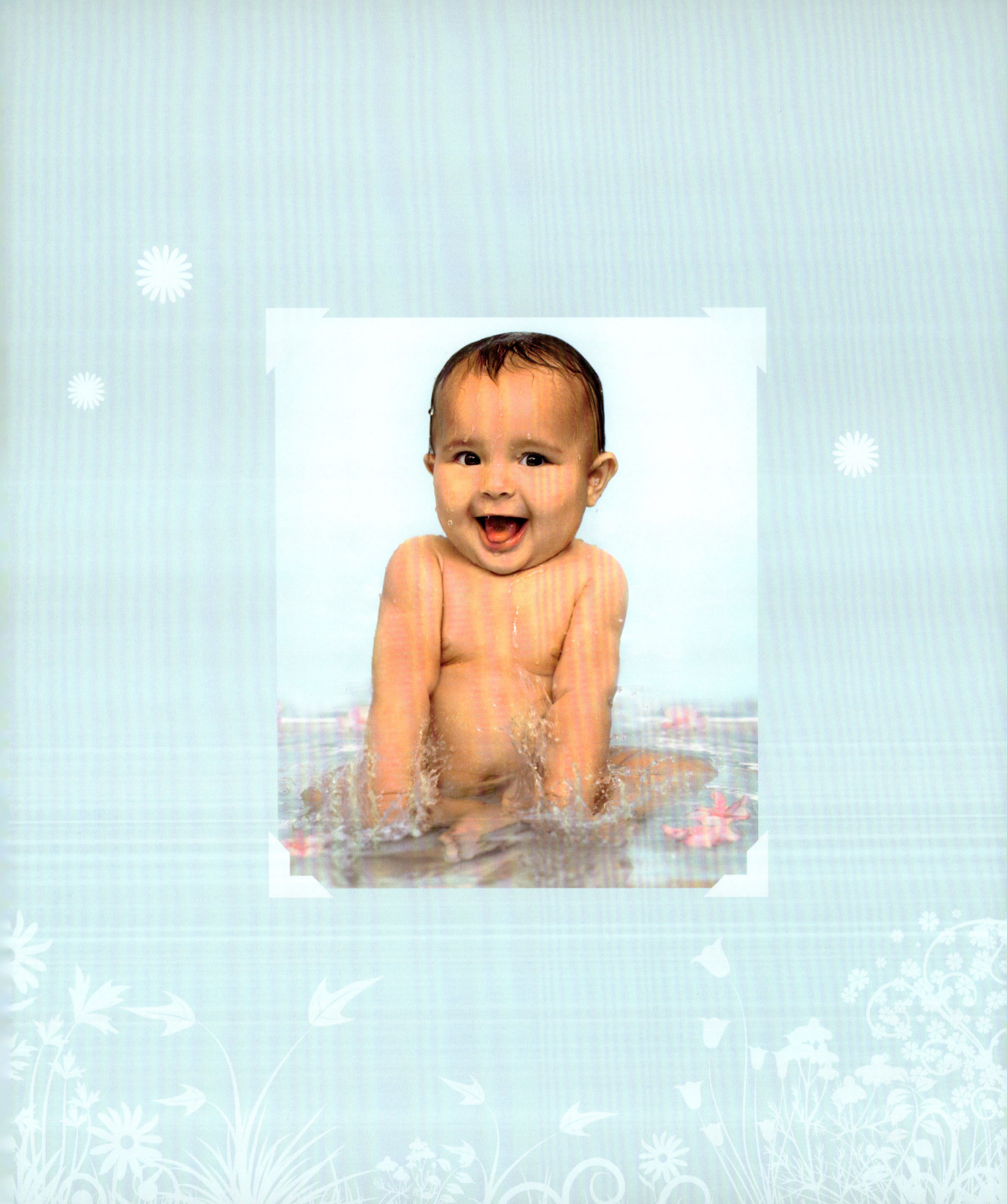

BATH TIME & WATERPLAY

MY FEELINGS
ABOUT BATH TIME

_____
_____
_____
_____

MY FAVOURITE
BATH TOY/S

_____
_____
_____
_____

WATER GAMES
I LOVE

_____
_____
_____

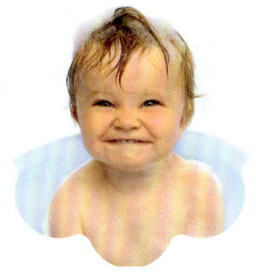

YOUR PHOTO HERE

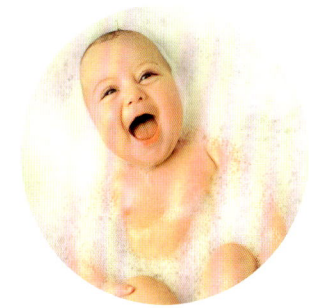

YOUR PHOTO HERE

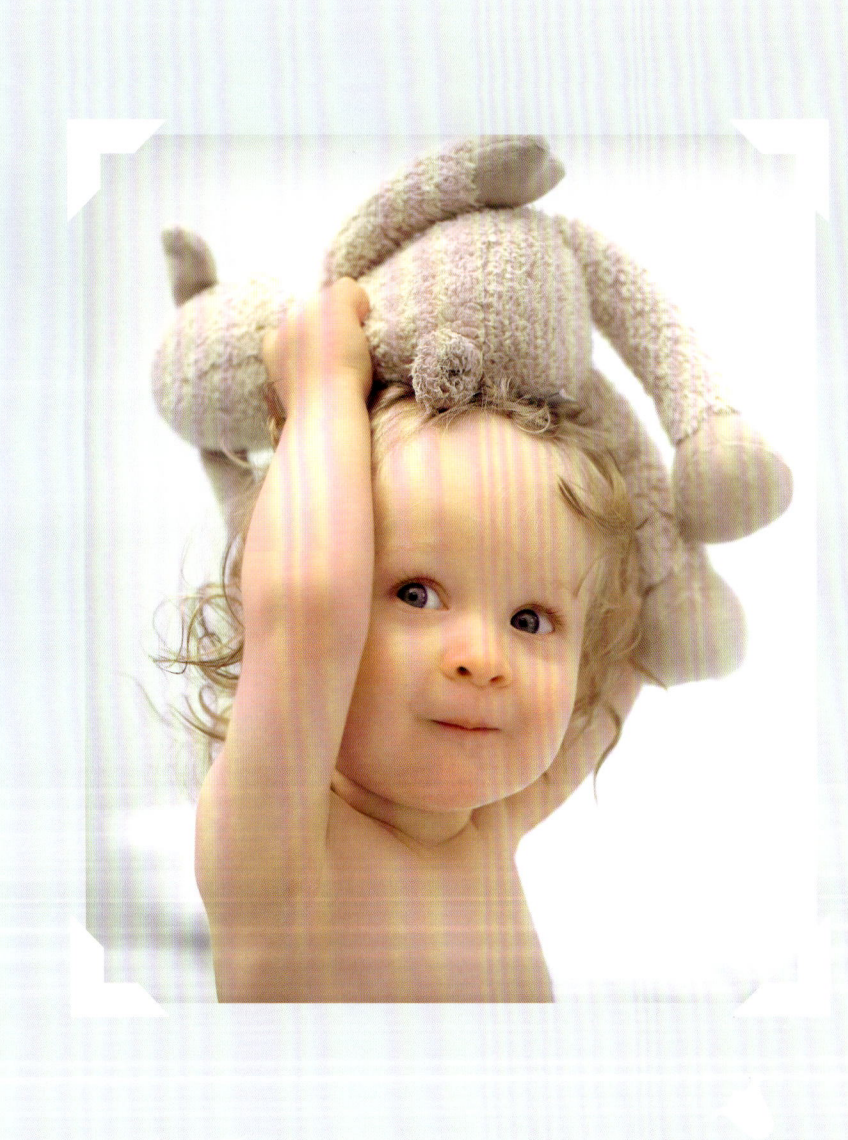

MY FAVOURITE THINGS

GAMES
_____

_____

_____

_____

TOYS
_____

_____

_____

BOOKS
_____

_____

_____

CLOTHES
_____

_____

_____

ACTIVITES
_____

_____

_____

PLACES
_____

_____

_____

_____

DRESS-UPS
_____

_____

_____

TELEVISION CHARACTERS
_____

_____

_____

COLOURS

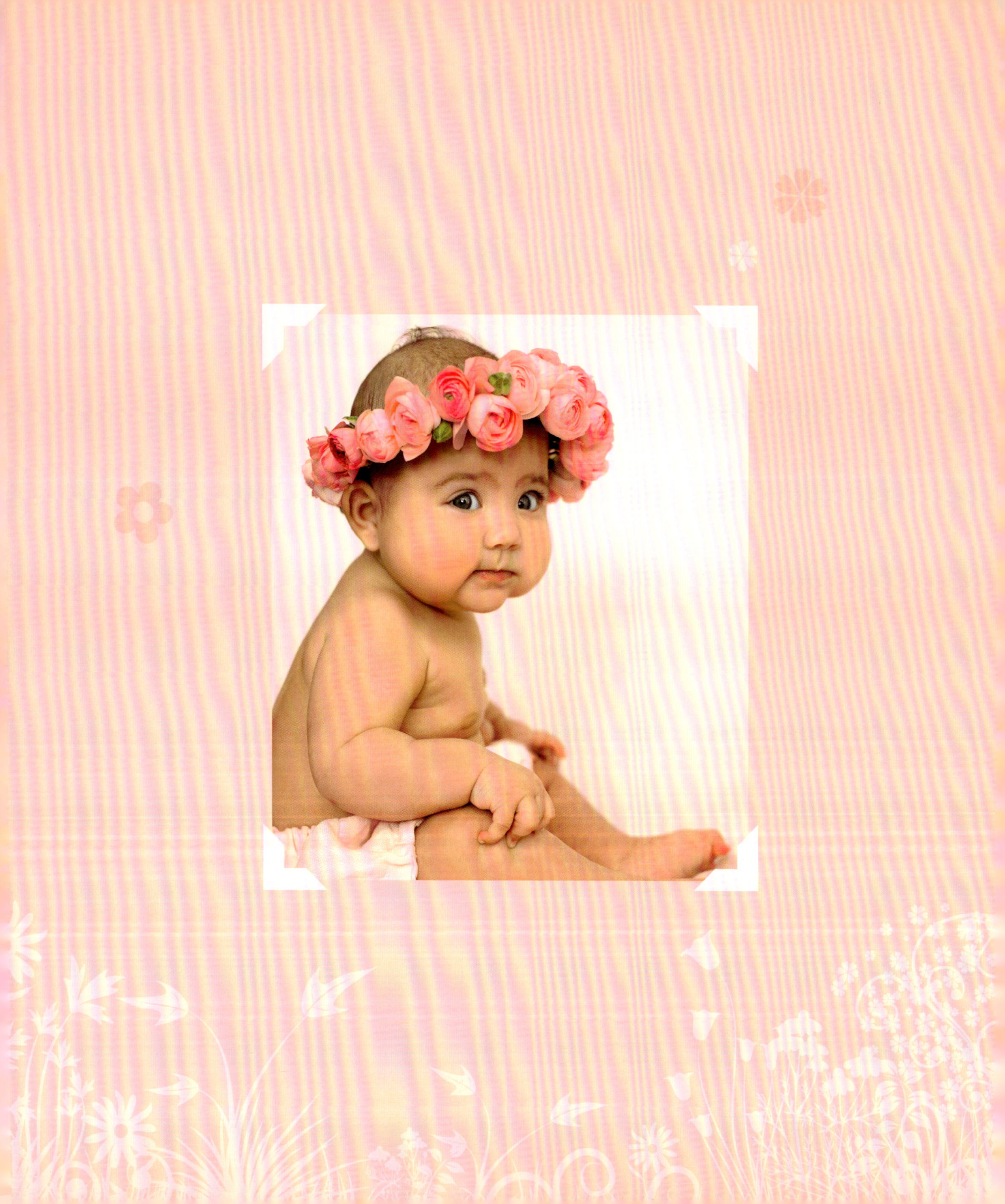

HOLIDAYS & TRAVEL

MY FIRST HOLIDAY

_____

_____

DATE

_____

WHERE WE WENT

_____

_____

WHO WENT WITH ME

_____

_____

_____

WHAT WE DID

_____

_____

_____

_____

_____

YOUR PHOTO HERE

YOUR PHOTO HERE

YOUR PHOTO HERE

YOUR PHOTO HERE

PHOTOGRAPHS

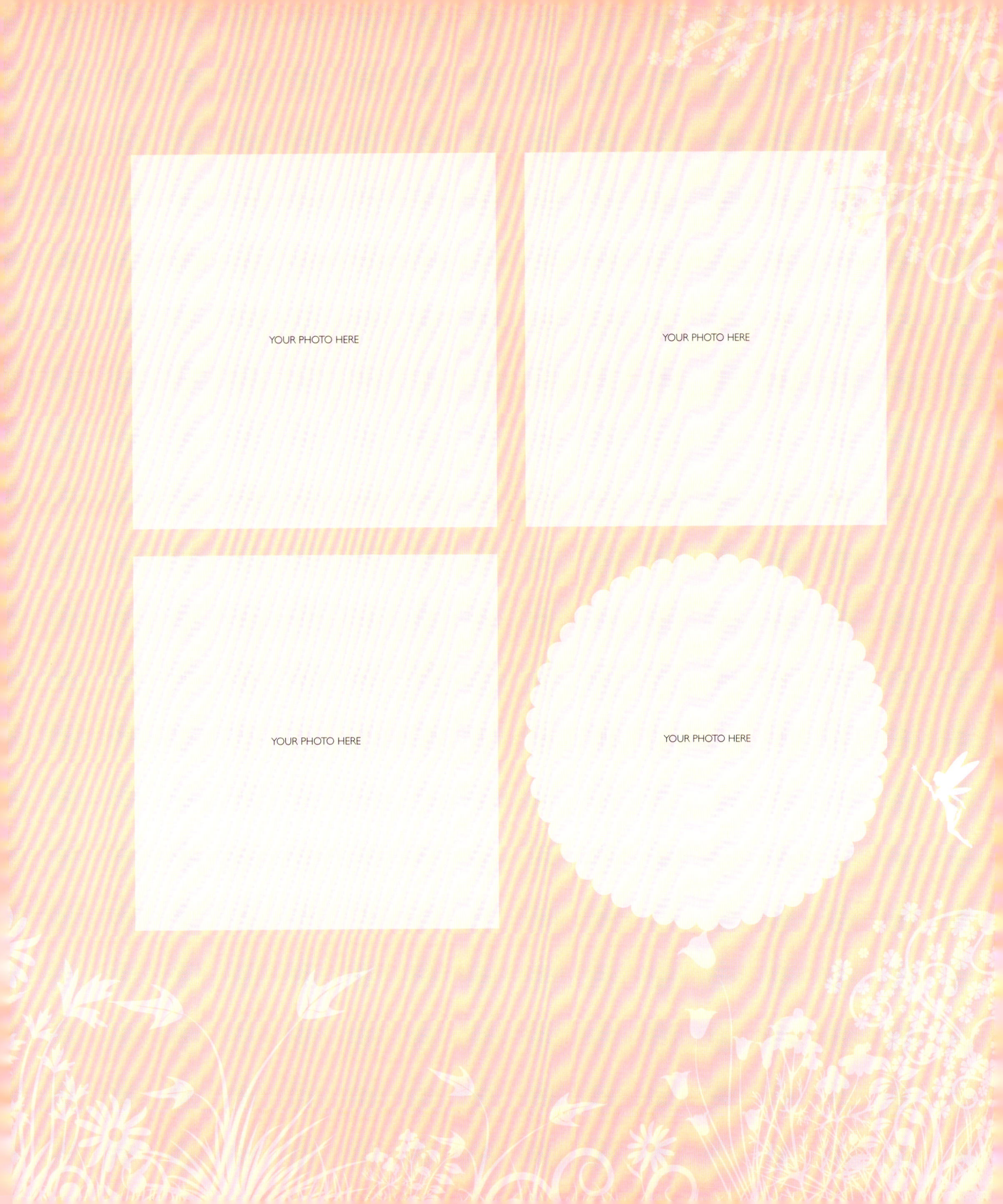

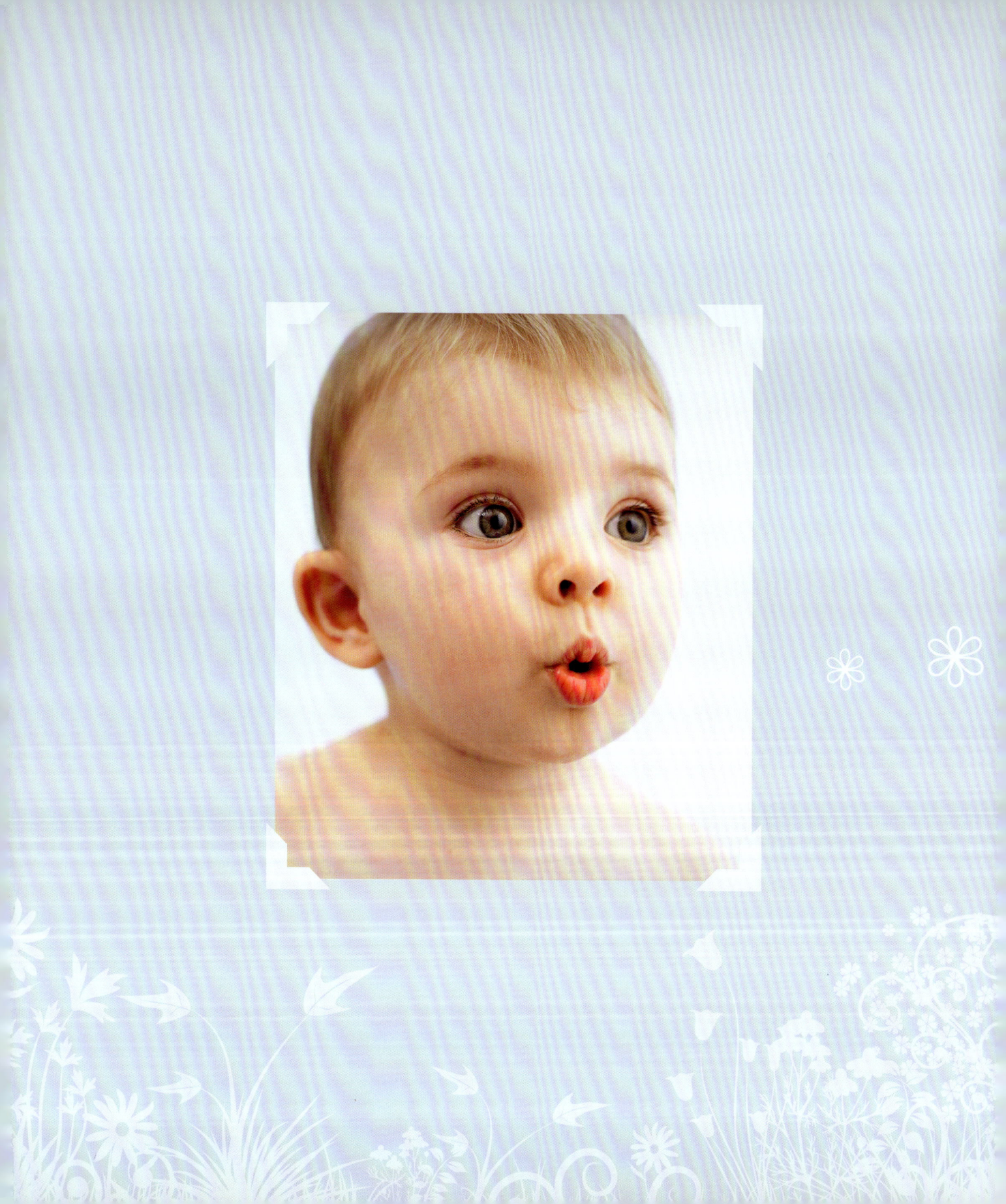

CELEBRATIONS & SPECIAL OCCASIONS

DATE

EVENT

FAMILY AND FRIENDS
WHO ATTENDED

DATE

EVENT

FAMILY AND FRIENDS
WHO ATTENDED

YOUR PHOTO HERE

YOUR PHOTO HERE

YOUR PHOTO HERE

YOUR PHOTO HERE

PHOTOGRAPHS

YOUR PHOTO HERE

YOUR PHOTO HERE

YOUR PHOTO HERE

YOUR PHOTO HERE

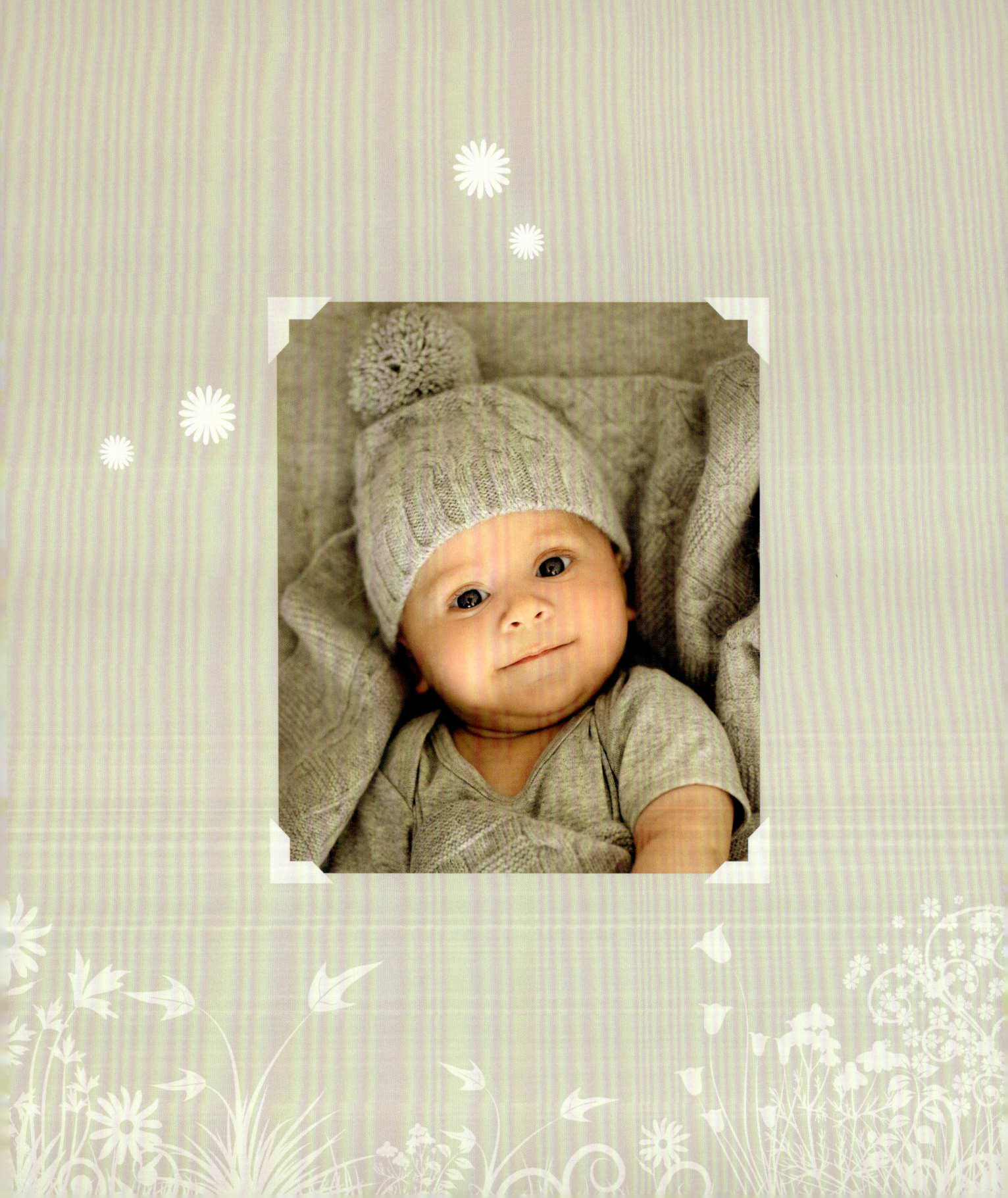

MY CAREGIVER/S NAMES

_____

_____

_____

WHERE THEY LOOK
AFTER ME

_____

_____

_____

GAMES THEY PLAY
WITH ME

_____

_____

_____

_____

_____

PICTURE

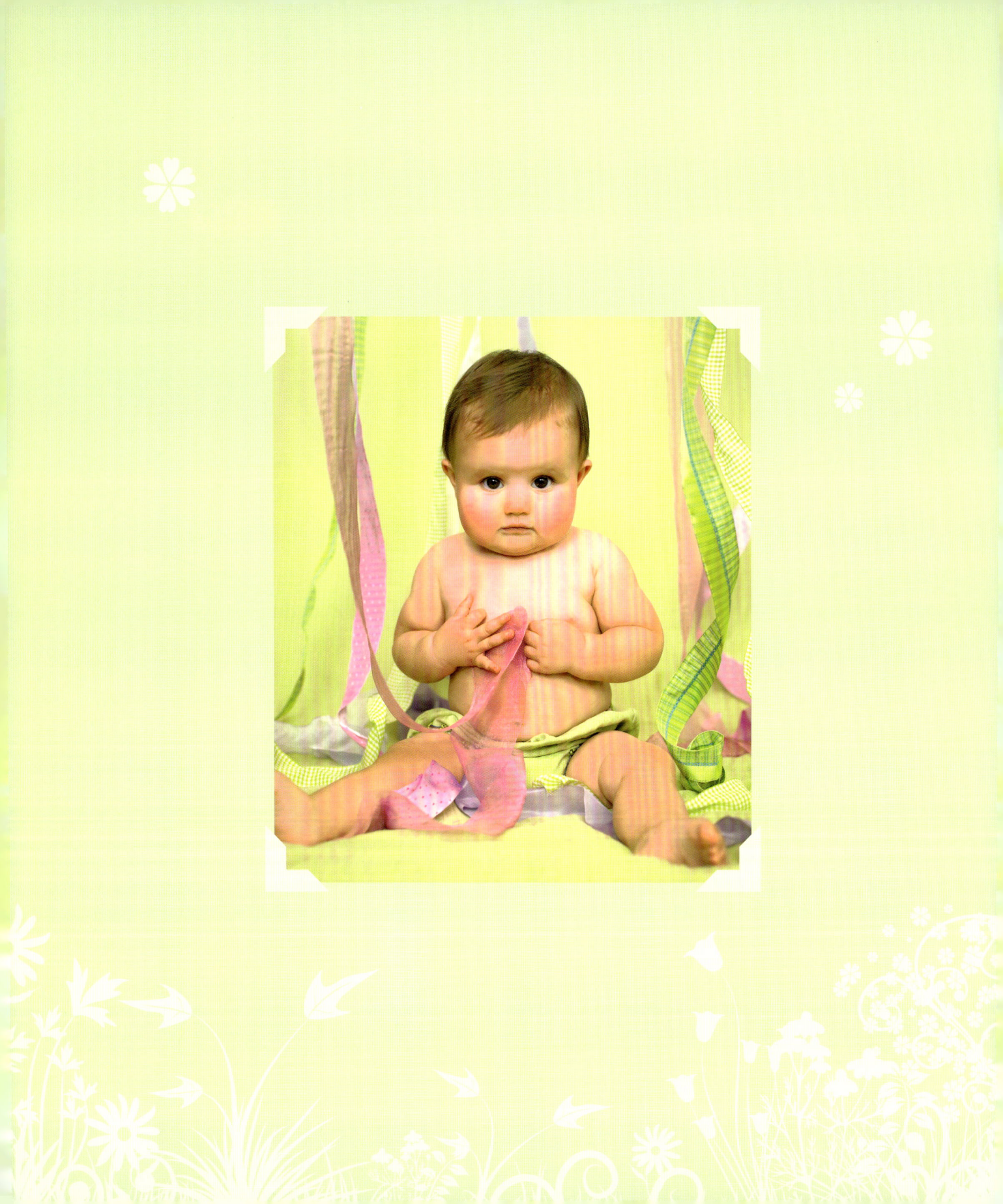

MY FIRST YEAR

MY FAVOURITE THINGS

GAMES _____

TOYS _____

BOOKS _____

ACTIVITIES _____

CLOTHES _____

COLOURS _____

TELEVISION CHARACTERS _____

PLACES _____

OTHER _____

_____

GOING OUT

FUN PLACES WE VISIT _____

_____

FAVOURITE OUTSIDE ACTIVITIES _____

_____

SPECIAL OUTINGS WITH GRANDPARENTS/RELATIVES/FRIENDS AND PLAYMATES _____

_____

_____

_____

YOUR PHOTO HERE

YOUR PHOTO HERE

YOUR PHOTO HERE

YOUR PHOTO HERE

MY FIRST BIRTHDAY PARTY

HOW WE CELEBRATED _____

_____

_____

_____

WHO ATTENDED _____

_____

_____

_____

_____

_____

_____

_____

_____

_____

_____

MY BIRTHDAY CAKE _____

_____

_____

MY FAVOURITE GIFT _____

_____

MY BIRTHDAY CAKE

YOUR PHOTO HERE

MY FAVOURITE GIFT

YOUR PHOTO HERE

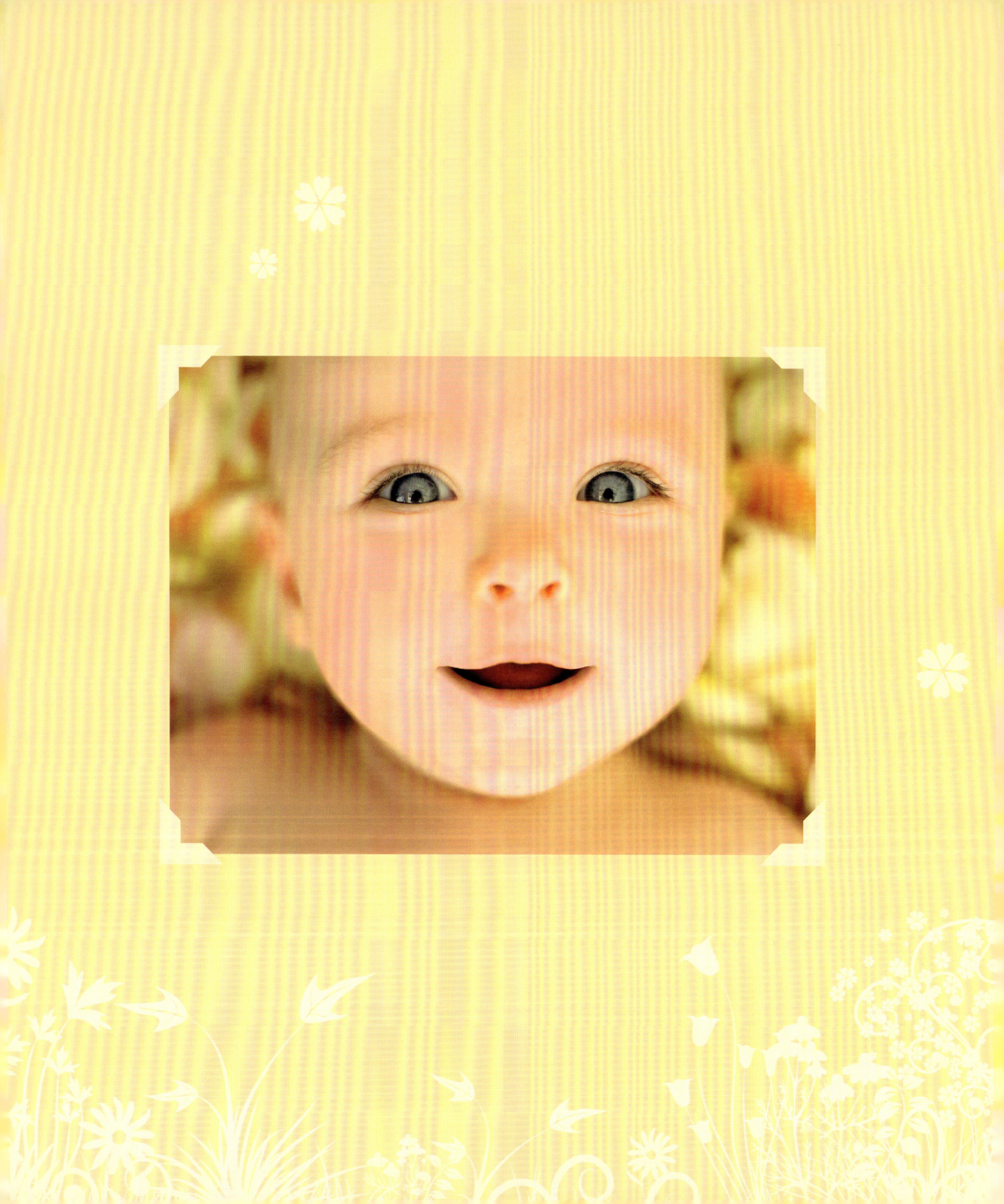

MY SECOND YEAR

MY FAVOURITE THINGS

GAMES

TOYS

BOOKS

ACTIVITIES

CLOTHES

COLOURS

TELEVISION CHARACTERS

PLACES

OTHER

GOING OUT

FUN PLACES WE VISIT

FAVOURITE OUTSIDE ACTIVITIES

SPECIAL OUTINGS WITH GRANDPARENTS/RELATIVES/FRIENDS AND PLAYMATES

YOUR PHOTO HERE

YOUR PHOTO HERE

YOUR PHOTO HERE

YOUR PHOTO HERE

PHOTOGRAPHS

MY SECOND BIRTHDAY PARTY

HOW WE CELEBRATED
_____
_____
_____
_____

WHO ATTENDED
_____
_____
_____
_____
_____
_____
_____
_____
_____
_____
_____

MY BIRTHDAY CAKE
_____
_____

MY FAVOURITE GIFT
_____
_____

MY BIRTHDAY CAKE

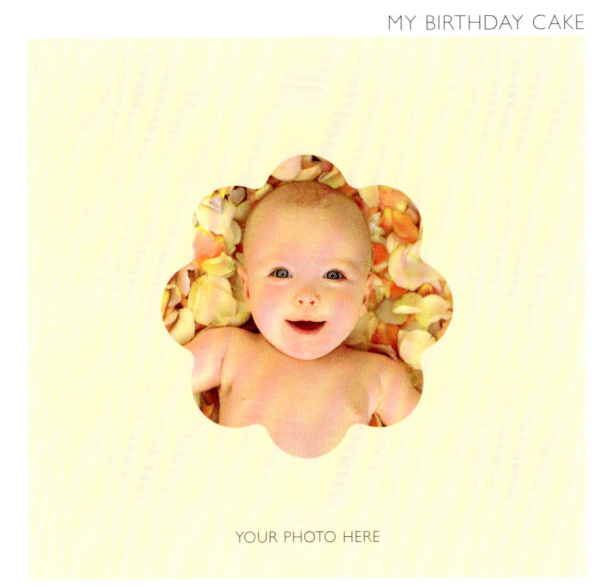

YOUR PHOTO HERE

MY FAVOURITE GIFT

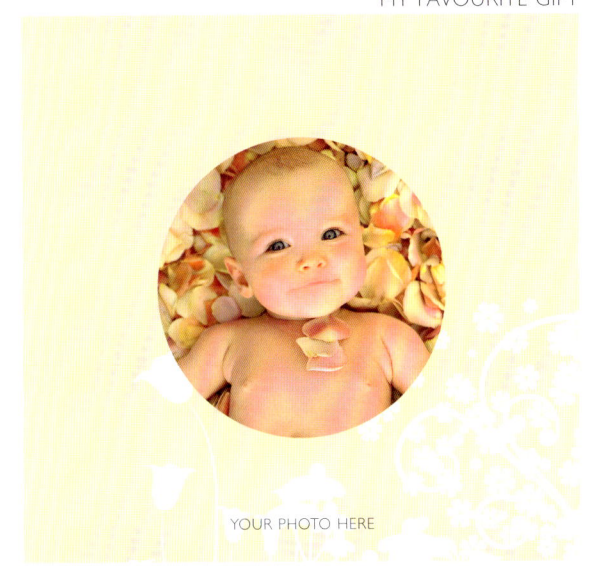

YOUR PHOTO HERE

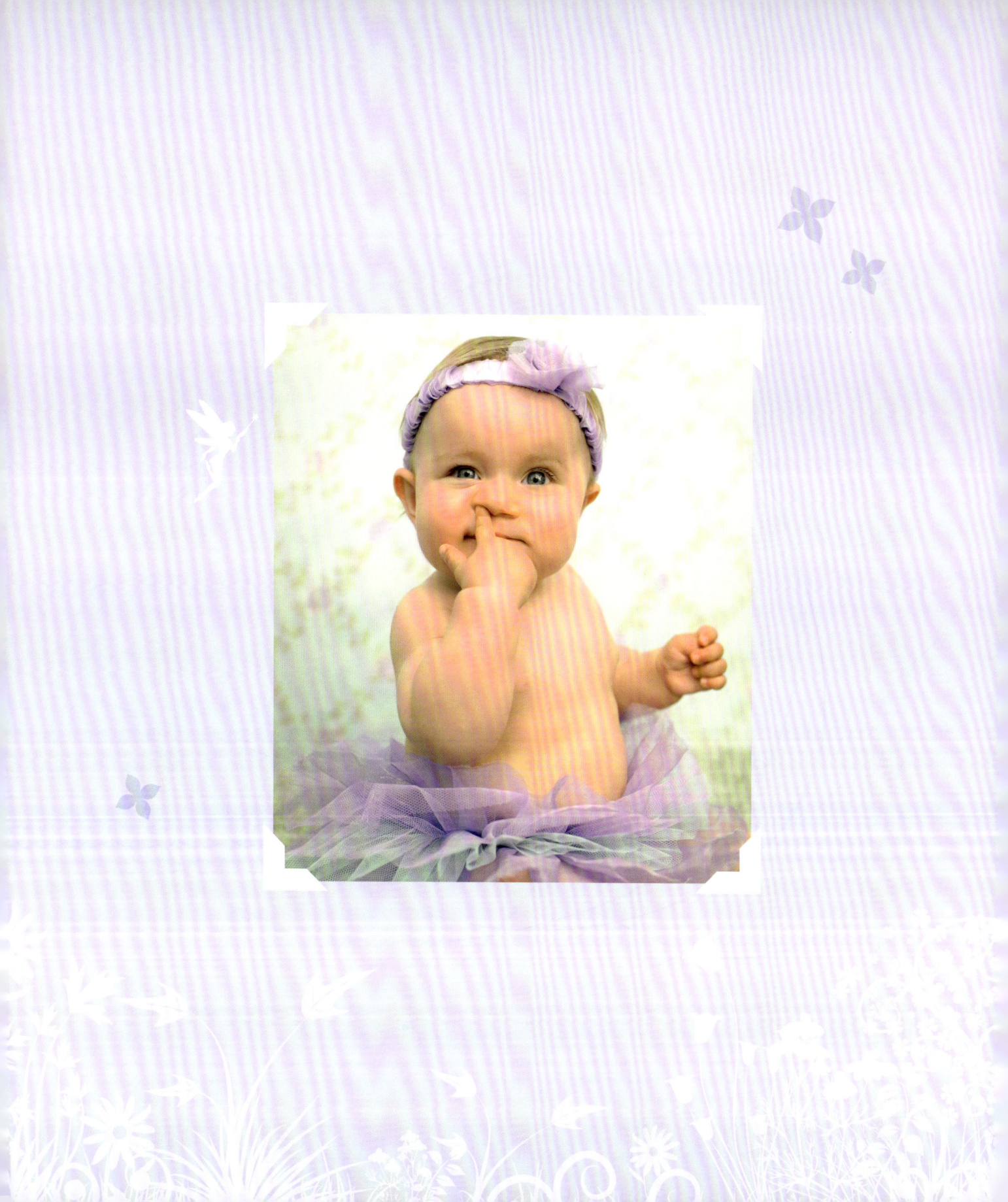

MY FAVOURITE THINGS

GAMES

TOYS

BOOKS

ACTIVITIES

CLOTHES

COLOURS

TELEVISION CHARACTERS

PLACES

OTHER

GOING OUT

FUN PLACES WE VISIT

FAVOURITE OUTSIDE ACTIVITIES

SPECIAL OUTINGS WITH GRANDPARENTS/RELATIVES/FRIENDS AND PLAYMATES

YOUR PHOTO HERE

YOUR PHOTO HERE

YOUR PHOTO HERE

YOUR PHOTO HERE

PHOTOGRAPHS

MY THIRD BIRTHDAY PARTY

HOW WE CELEBRATED

_____

_____

_____

WHO ATTENDED

_____

_____

_____

_____

_____

_____

_____

_____

MY BIRTHDAY CAKE

_____

_____

MY FAVOURITE GIFT

_____

MY BIRTHDAY CAKE

YOUR PHOTO HERE

MY FAVOURITE GIFT

YOUR PHOTO HERE

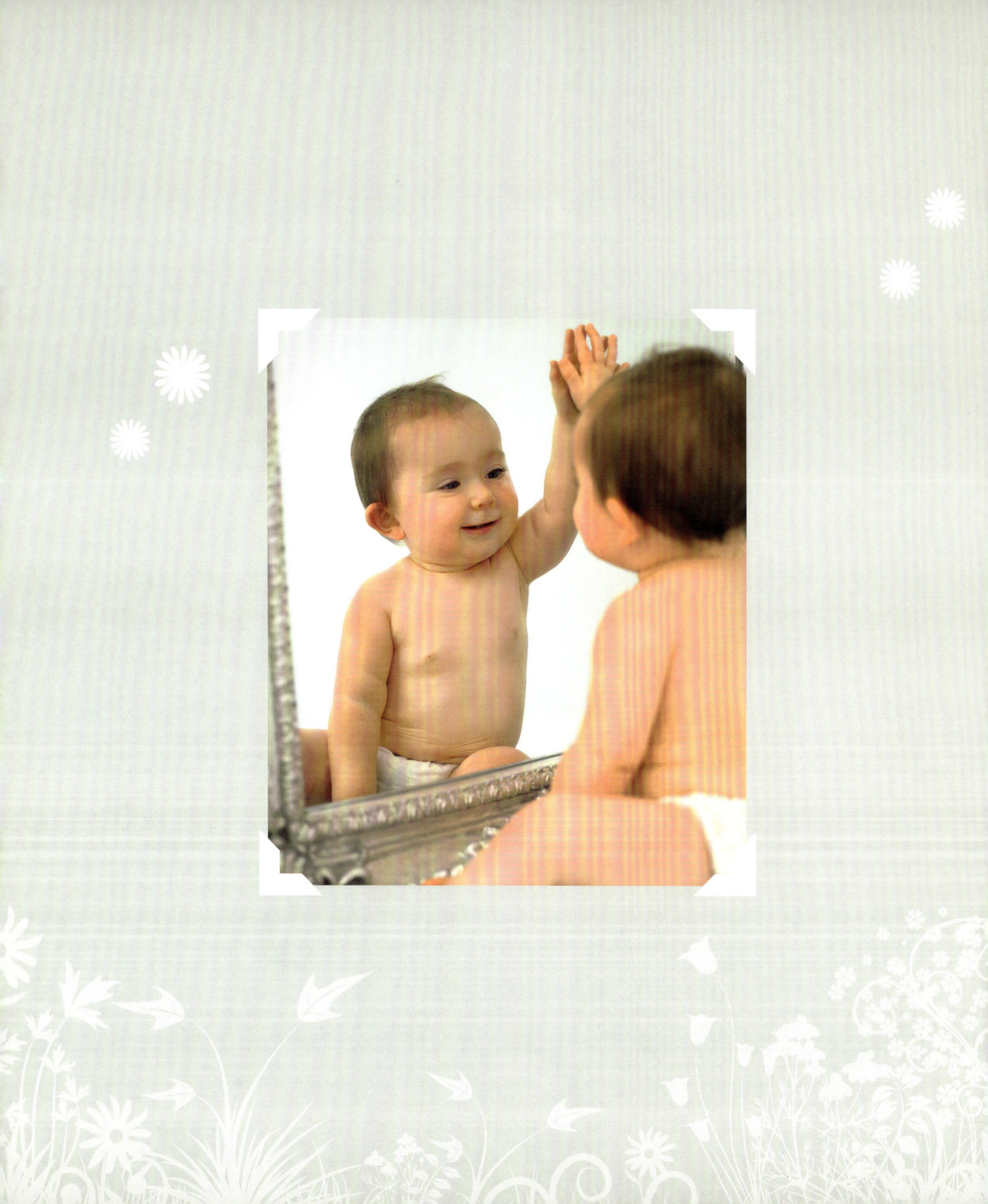

MY FAVOURITE THINGS

GAMES

TOYS

BOOKS

ACTIVITIES

CLOTHES

COLOURS

TELEVISION CHARACTERS

PLACES

OTHER

GOING OUT

FUN PLACES WE VISIT

FAVOURITE OUTSIDE ACTIVITIES

SPECIAL OUTINGS WITH GRANDPARENTS/RELATIVES/FRIENDS AND PLAYMATES

YOUR PHOTO HERE

YOUR PHOTO HERE

YOUR PHOTO HERE

YOUR PHOTO HERE

PHOTOGRAPHS

HOW WE CELEBRATED
_____
_____
_____
_____

WHO ATTENDED
_____
_____
_____
_____
_____
_____
_____
_____
_____
_____

MY BIRTHDAY CAKE
_____
_____
_____

MY FAVOURITE GIFT
_____

MY BIRTHDAY CAKE

YOUR PHOTO HERE

MY FAVOURITE GIFT

YOUR PHOTO HERE

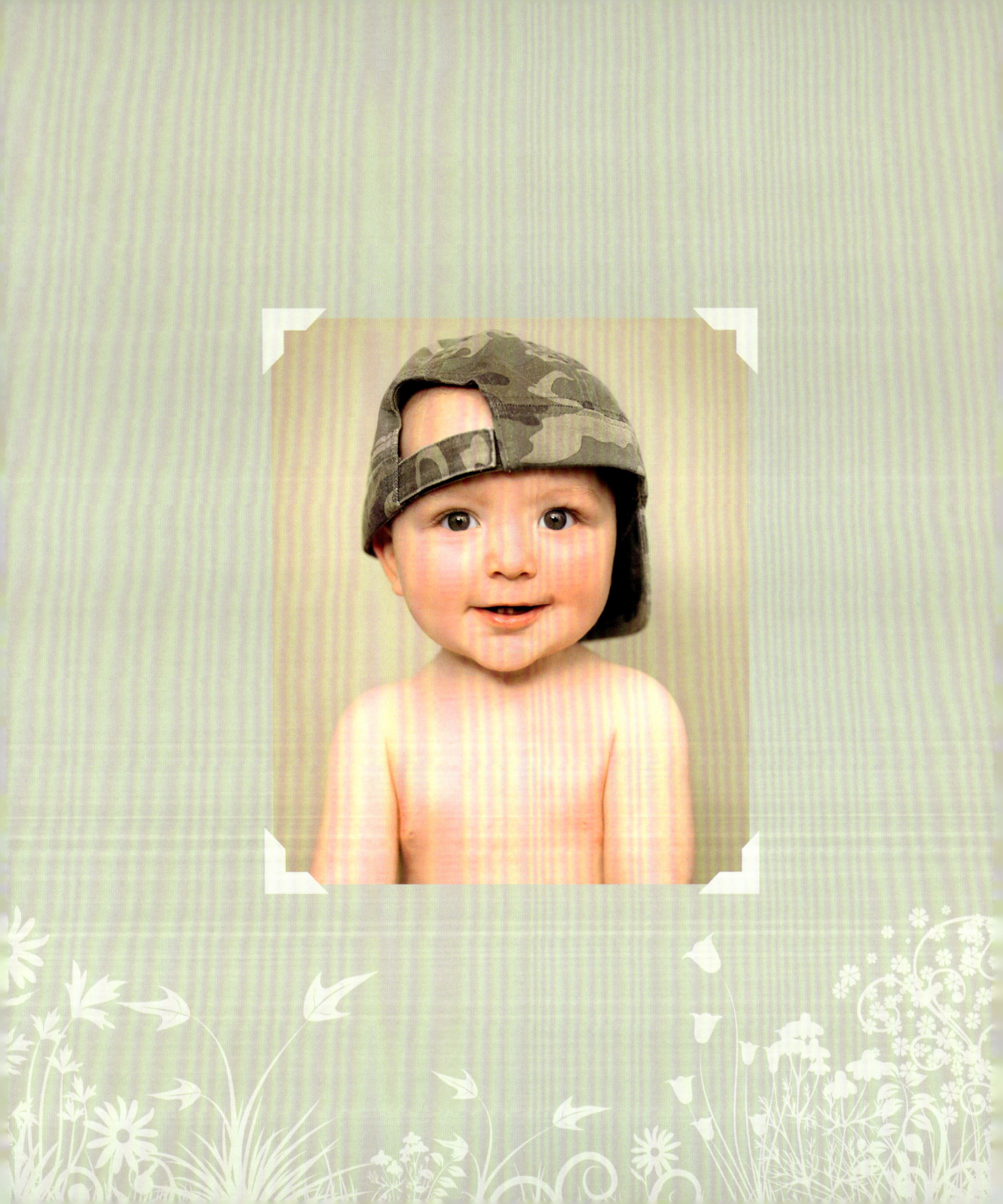

MY FIFTH YEAR

MY FAVOURITE THINGS

GAMES

TOYS

BOOKS

ACTIVITIES

CLOTHES

COLOURS

TELEVISION CHARACTERS

PLACES

OTHER

GOING OUT

FUN PLACES WE VISIT

FAVOURITE OUTSIDE ACTIVITIES

SPECIAL OUTINGS WITH GRANDPARENTS/RELATIVES/FRIENDS AND PLAYMATES

YOUR PHOTO HERE

YOUR PHOTO HERE

YOUR PHOTO HERE

YOUR PHOTO HERE

PHOTOGRAPHS

MY FIFTH BIRTHDAY PARTY

HOW WE CELEBRATED

_____

_____

_____

WHO ATTENDED

_____

_____

_____

_____

_____

_____

_____

_____

MY BIRTHDAY CAKE

_____

_____

MY FAVOURITE GIFT

_____

MY BIRTHDAY CAKE

YOUR PHOTO HERE

MY FAVOURITE GIFT

YOUR PHOTO HERE

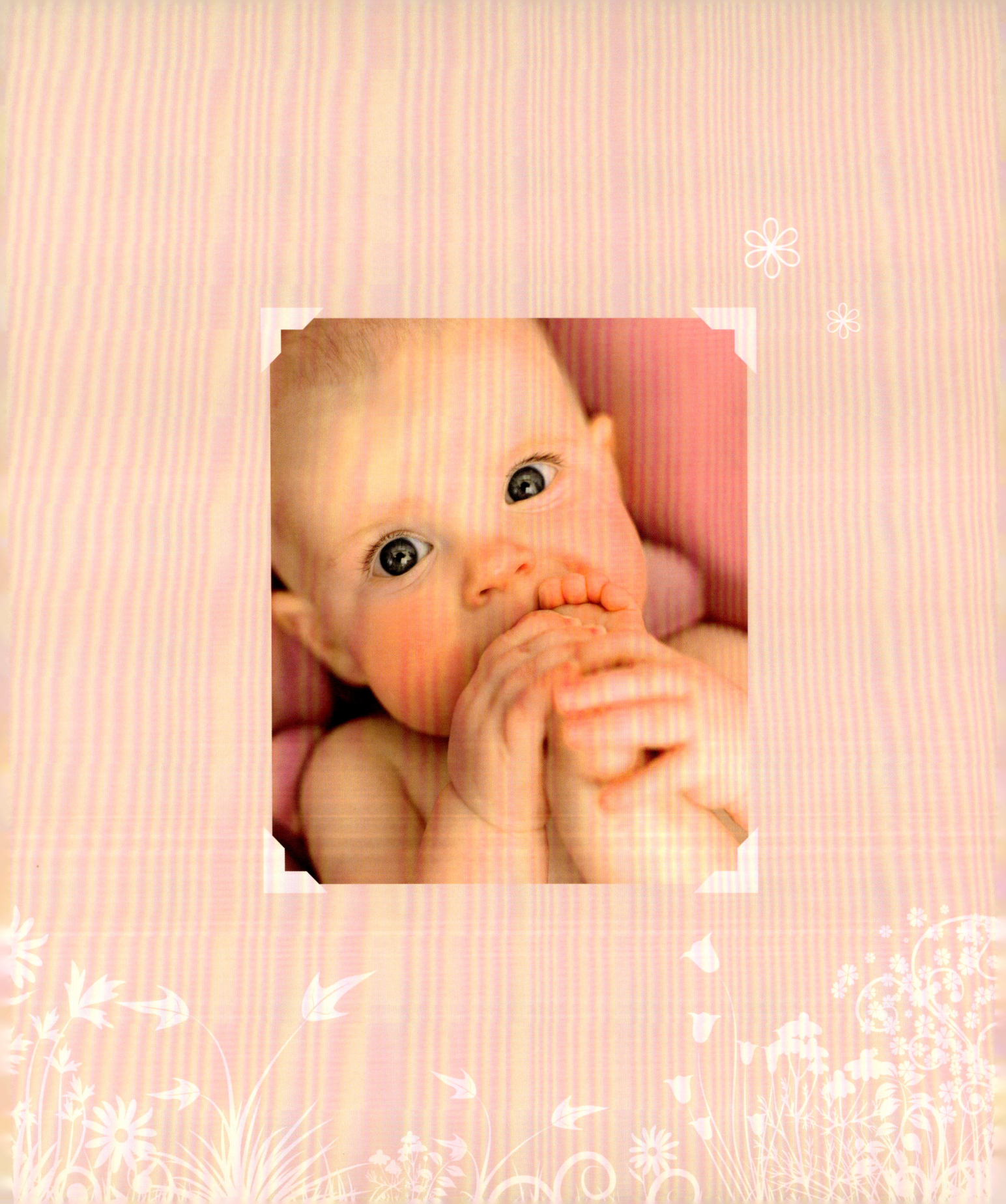

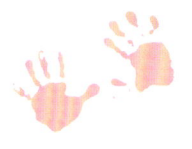

HAND & FOOT PRINTS

IN THE BEGINNING

DATE _____

HAND

FOOT

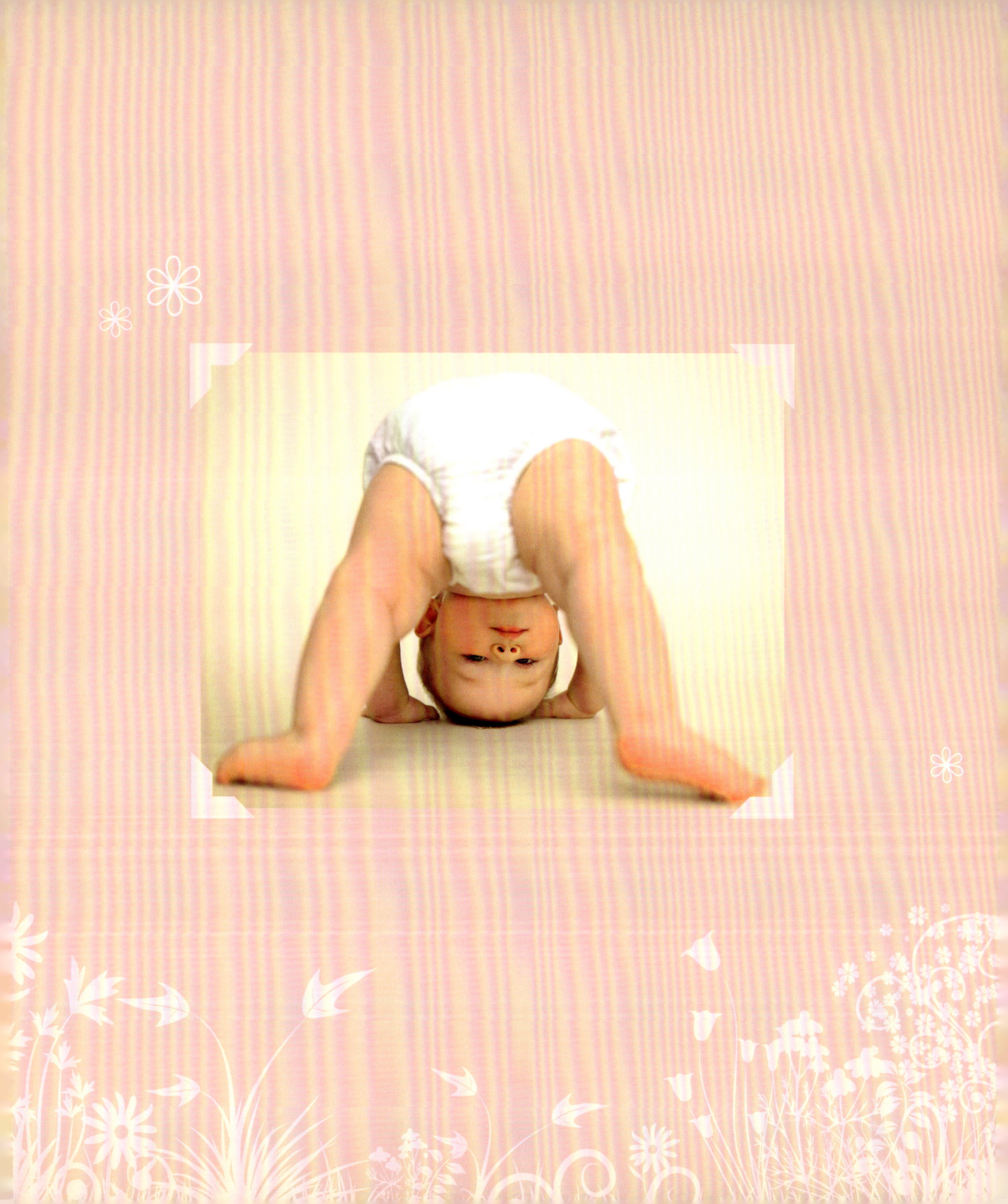

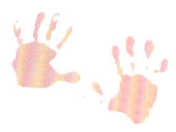

HAND & FOOT PRINTS
AT AGE FIVE

DATE _____

HAND

FOOT

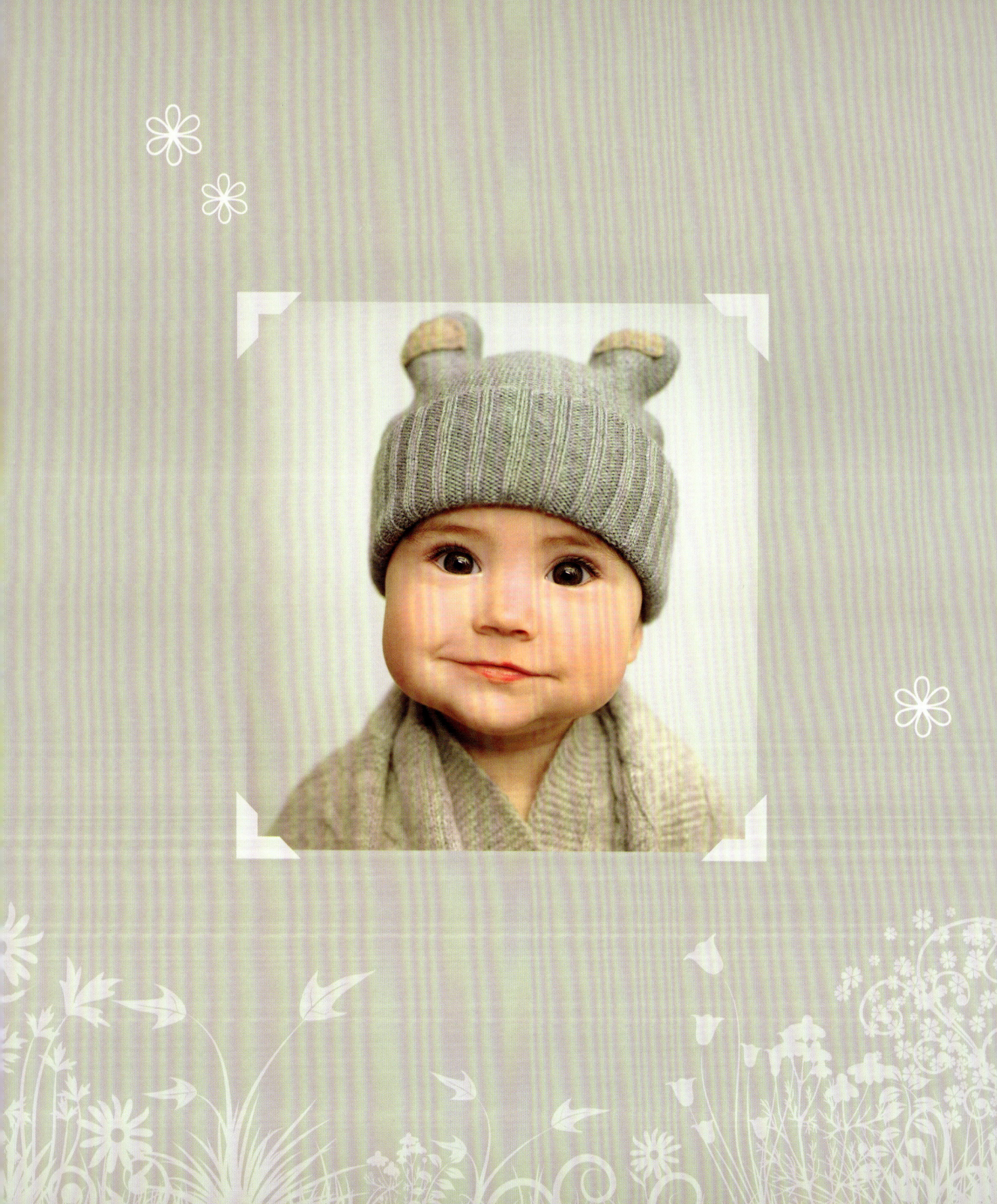

HEALTH

BLOOD TYPE

_____

ALLERGIES

_____

_____

_____

_____

IMMUNISATION	AGE	DATE

ILLNESSES	AGE	DATE

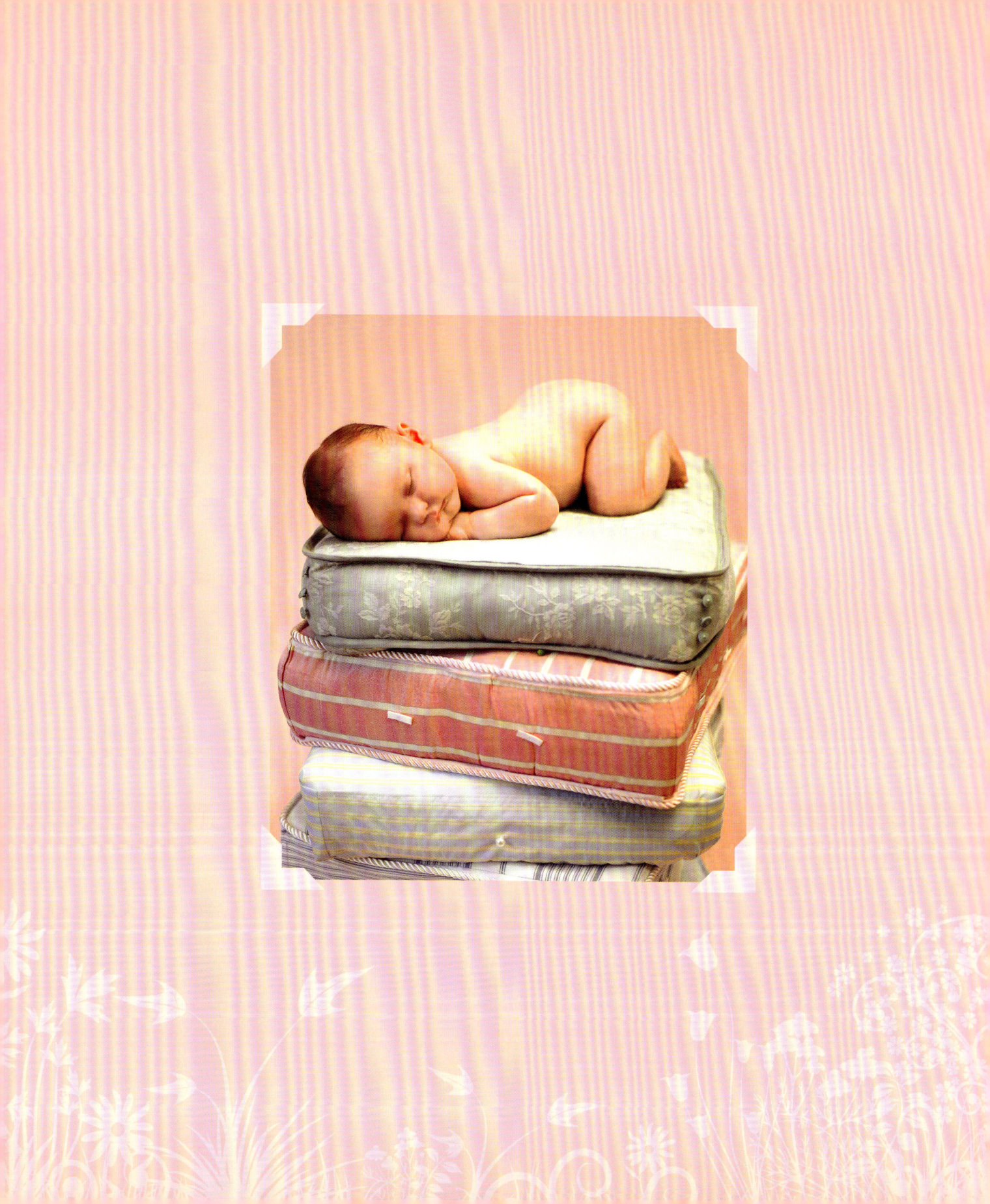

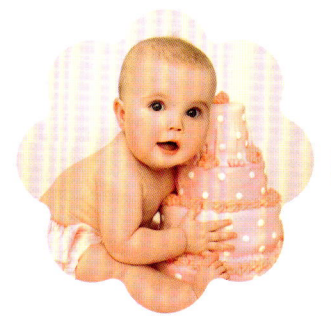

GROWTH

HEIGHT

BORN

3MTHS

6MTHS

9MTHS

1YR

2YR

3YR

4YR

5YR

MY HEIGHT CHART

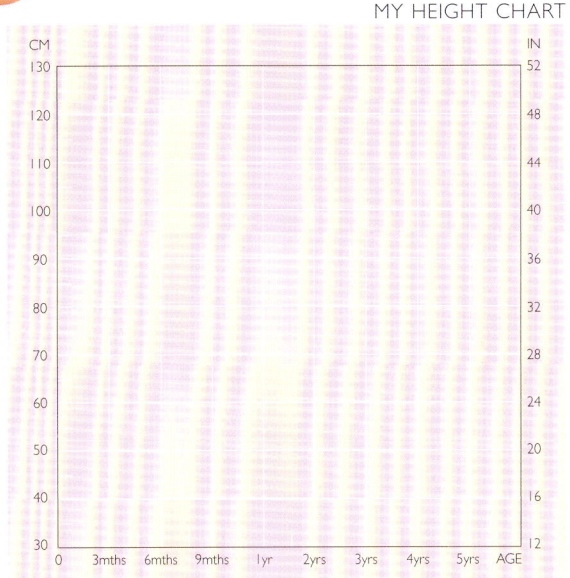

WEIGHT

BORN

3MTHS

6MTHS

9MTHS

1YR

2YR

3YR

4YR

5YR

MY WEIGHT CHART

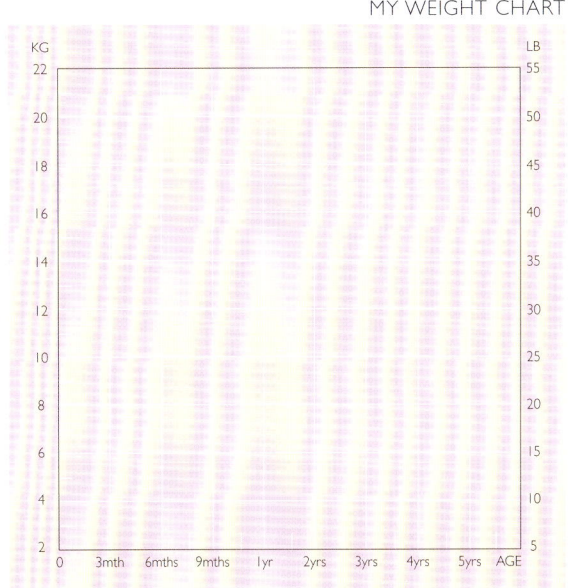

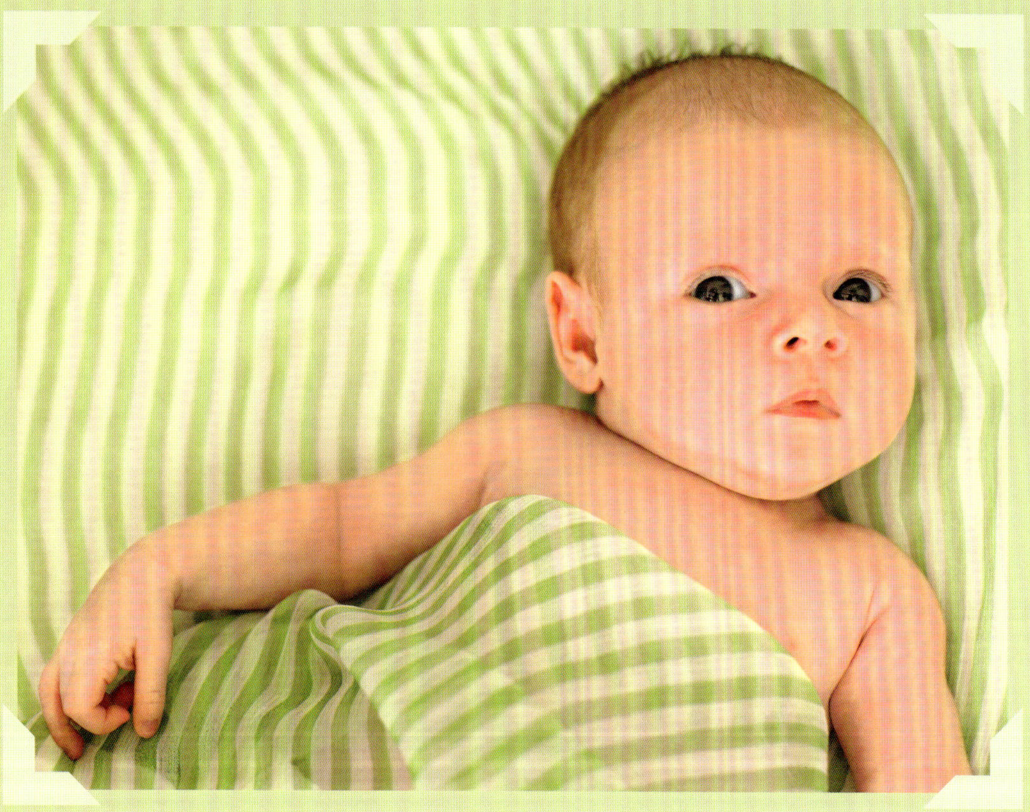

MY PARENTS' SPECIAL
MESSAGE FOR ME

DATE

MILESTONES

DATE

MY FIRST TOOTH

MY FIRST TOOTHBRUSH

MY FIRST BED

MY FIRST NIGHT AWAY FROM HOME

MY FIRST WORD

MY FIRST STEP

MY FIRST DAY AT PRESCHOOL

MY FIRST DAY AT SCHOOL

MY FIRST SHOES

I WAS   OLD

THEY WERE SIZE

MY FIRST HAIRCUT

I WAS   OLD

CUT BY

MY FIRST FRIEND

MY FIRST PET

MY FIRST BICYCLE

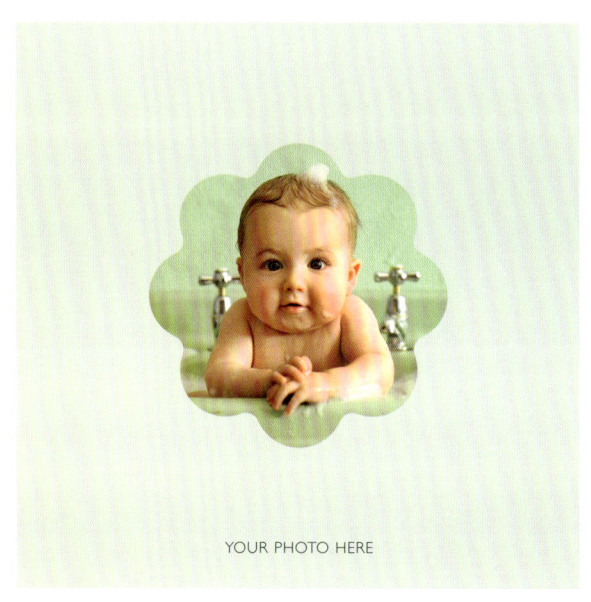

YOUR PHOTO HERE

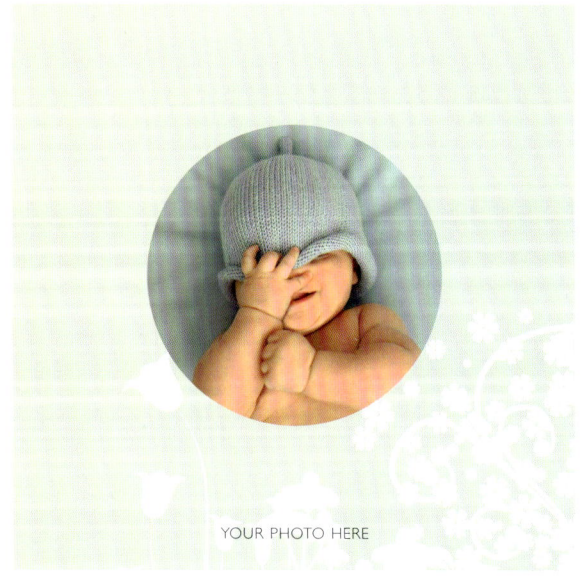

YOUR PHOTO HERE

The Five Mile Press Pty Ltd
1 Centre Road, Scoresby
Victoria 3179 Australia
www.fivemile.com.au

ISBN: 978-1-74211-029-5

This edition produced and originated by PQ Blackwell Limited,
116 Symonds Street, Auckland, New Zealand
www.pqblackwell.com

First published in 2008. This edition published in 2009 by The Five Mile Press Pty Ltd.

Printed by 1010 Printing Ltd, China 5 4 3